Obesity Management

Guest Editors

ANN RODDEN, DO, MS
VANESSA DIAZ, MD, MS

PRIMARY CARE:
CLINICS IN OFFICE PRACTICE

www.primarycare.theclinics.com

Consulting Editor
JOEL J. HEIDELBAUGH, MD

June 2009 • Volume 36 • Number 2

SAUNDERS an imprint of ELSEVIER, Inc.

W.B. SAUNDERS COMPANY
A Division of Elsevier Inc.

1600 John F. Kennedy Boulevard, Suite 1800 • Philadelphia, PA 19103-2899

http://www.theclinics.com

PRIMARY CARE: CLINICS IN OFFICE PRACTICE Volume 36, Number 2
June 2009 ISSN 0095-4543, ISBN-13: 978-1-4377-0533-1, ISBN-10: 1-4377-0533-2

Editor: Barbara Cohen-Kligerman
Developmental Editor: Theresa Collier

Primary Care: Clinics in Office Practice (ISSN: 0095–4543) is published quarterly by Elsevier Inc., 360 Park Avenue South, New York, NY 10010-1710. Months of issue are March, June, September, and December. Business and Editorial Offices: 1600 John F. Kennedy Blvd., Suite 1800, Philadelphia, PA 19103-2899. Customer Service Office: 6277 Sea Harbor Drive, Orlando, FL 32887–4800. Periodicals postage paid at New York, NY and additional mailing offices. Subscription prices are $176.00 per year (US individuals), $296.00 (US institutions), $89.00 (US students), $215.00 (Canadian individuals), $348.00 (Canadian institutions), $140.00 (Canadian students), $268.00 (foreign individuals), $348.00 (foreign institutions), and $140.00 (foreign students). Foreign air speed delivery is included in all *Clinics* subscription prices. All prices are subject to change without notice. POSTMASTER: Send address changes to *Primary Care: Clinics in Office Practice*, Elsevier Periodicals Customer Service, 11830 Westline Industrial Drive, St. Louis, MO 63146. Customer Service (orders, claims, online, change of address): Elsevier Periodicals Customer Service, 11830 Westline Industrial Drive, St. Louis, MO 63146. Tel: 1-800-654-2452 (U.S. and Canada); 314-453-7041 (outside U.S. and Canada). Fax: 314-453-5170. E-mail: journalscustomerservice-usa@elsevier.com (for print support); journalsonlinesupport-usa@elsevier.com (for online support).

Reprints. For copies of 100 or more, of articles in this publication, please contact the Commercial Reprints Department, Elsevier Inc., 360 Park Avenue South, New York, NY 10010-1710. Tel. (212) 633-3812; Fax: (212) 482-1935; E-mail: reprints@elsevier.com.

Primary Care: Clinics in Office Practice is covered in *MEDLINE/PubMed (Index Medicus) and EMBASE/Excerpta Medica, Current Contents/Clinical Medicine, and ISI/BIOMED.*

Printed in the United States of America.

Contributors

CONSULTING EDITOR

JOEL J. HEIDELBAUGH, MD
Clinical Assistant Professor, Departments of Family Medicine and Urology; Clerkship Director, Department of Family Medicine, University of Michigan Medical School, Ann Arbor; Ypsilanti Health Center, Ypsilanti, Michigan

GUEST EDITORS

ANN RODDEN, DO, MS
Assistant Professor, Department of Family Medicine, Medical University of South Carolina, Charleston, South Carolina

VANESSA DIAZ, MD, MS
Assistant Professor, Department of Family Medicine, Medical University of South Carolina, Charleston, South Carolina

AUTHORS

ADRIENNE ABLES, PharmD
Associate Professor of Family Medicine, Medical University of South Carolina, Spartanburg Family Medicine Residency, Spartanburg, South Carolina

PAULA ANDERSON-WORTS, DO, MPH
Associate Professor of Family Medicine and Public Health, Department of Family Medicine and Public Health, Nova Southeastern University College of Osteopathic Medicine, Davie, Florida

MEGAN K. BAKER, MD
Assistant Professor of Surgery, Department of Surgery, Medical University of South Carolina, Charleston, South Carolina

MARK N. BEARD, MD
University of Missouri, Family Medicine Residency Program, Columbia, Missouri

DEBRA BOARDLEY, PhD, RD
Professor, Department of Public Health, College of Medicine, University of Toledo; Coordinator, MPH–Public Health Nutrition, Northwest Ohio Consortium for Public Health, Toledo, Ohio

NATHAN F. BRADFORD, MD
AnMed Family Medicine Residency Program, Anderson, South Carolina

T. KARL BYRNE, MD
Professor of Surgery, Department of Surgery, Medical University of South Carolina, Charleston, South Carolina

PABLO J. CALZADA, DO, MPH, FAAFP
Assistant Dean of Clinical Operations; Department of Family Medicine and Public Health, Nova Southeastern University College of Osteopathic Medicine, Davie, Florida

PETER J. CAREK, MD, MS
Professor and Associate Residency Program Director, Department of Family Medicine, Medical University of South Carolina, Charleston, South Carolina

ESA DAVIS, MD, MPH
Assistant Professor, Department of Family Medicine, Case Western Reserve University, Cleveland, Ohio

LORI M. DICKERSON, PharmD, BCPS
Professor and Associate Residency Program Director, Department of Family Medicine, Medical University of South Carolina, Charleston, South Carolina

MARK E. FELDMANN, MD
Chief Resident, Department of Surgery, Medical University of South Carolina, Charleston, South Carolina

MARK K. HUNTINGTON, MD, PhD, FAAFP
Associate Professor, Department of Family Medicine, Sanford School of Medicine, University of South Dakota; Assistant Director, Sioux Falls Family Medicine Residency Program, Center for Family Medicine, Sioux Falls, South Dakota

PAUL V. JACKSON, MD
Assistant Clinical Professor of Family Medicine, Virginia Commonwealth University, St. Francis Family Medicine Residency Program, Midlothian, Virginia

RICHELLE J. KOOPMAN, MD, MS
Assistant Professor, Curtis W. and Ann H. Long Department of Family and Community Medicine, University of Missouri, Columbia, Missouri

MISTY M. MANN, MA
Argosy University, Chicago (Formerly the Illinois School of Professional Psychology), Chicago, Illinois

MAREK MARCINKIEWICZ, MD
PGY 2 Resident, Family Medicine, Virginia Commonwealth University, St. Francis Family Medicine Residency Program, Midlothian, Virginia

SUSAN E. MEADOWS, MLS
Medical Librarian; Adjunct Associate Professor, Information Management and Resource Center, Curtis W. and Ann H. Long Department of Family and Community Medicine, University of Missouri, Columbia, Missouri

DOUGLAS M. OKAY, MD
Assistant Clinical Professor of Family Medicine, Virginia Commonwealth University, St. Francis Family Medicine Residency Program, Midlothian, Virginia

CHRISTINE OLSON, PhD
Professor, Division of Nutritional Services, Cornell University, Ithaca, New York

M. NOVELLA PAPINO, MD
PGY 2 Resident, Family Medicine, Virginia Commonwealth University St. Francis Family Medicine Residency Program, Midlothian, Virginia

REBECCA S. POBOCIK, PhD, RD
Coordinator, MPH–Public Health Nutrition, Northwest Ohio Consortium for Public Health, Toledo; Associate Professor, Department of Nutrition, School of Family and Consumer Sciences, Bowling Green State University, Bowling Green, Ohio

KAVITHA BHAT SCHELBERT, MD, MS
Assistant Professor, Department of Family Medicine, University of Pittsburgh School of Medicine, Pittsburgh, Pennsylvania

ROGER A. SHEWMAKE, PhD, LN
Professor and Director, Section of Nutrition, Department of Family Medicine, Sanford School of Medicine, University of South Dakota; Sioux Falls Family Medicine Residency Program, Center for Family Medicine, Sioux Falls, South Dakota

TERRENCE E. STEYER, MD
Associate Professor, Department of Family Medicine, Medical University of South Carolina, Charleston, South Carolina

SARAH J. SWOFFORD, MD
Assistant Professor of Clinical Family and Community Medicine, Curtis W. and Ann H. Long Department of Family and Community Medicine, University of Missouri, Columbia, Missouri

MARY R. TALEN, PhD
Director of Behavioral Health Science, MacNeal Family Medicine Residency Program, Berwyn, Illinois

Contents

Foreword xiii

Joel J. Heidelbaugh

Preface xv

Ann Rodden and Vanessa Diaz

Obesity on the Rise 243

Debra Boardley and Rebecca S. Pobocik

The prevalence of obesity has increased markedly during recent years with the burden of obesity higher in minority groups in the United States. Rates of obesity vary according to age and employment, although the effect by socioeconomic strata is diminishing. Body mass index (BMI) and waist circumference (WC) are the primary anthropometric measures of obesity, but waist-to-height is increasingly being used as a measure that identifies both overweight and metabolic risk. BMI should be interpreted with caution in the elderly, children, and some Asian populations.

Obesity and Metabolic Disease 257

Richelle J. Koopman, Sarah J. Swofford, Mark N. Beard, and Susan E. Meadows

Obesity independently increases the risk of developing diabetes 10-fold compared with that for patients who are normal weight. Overweight patients with impaired glucose tolerance (IGT) or impaired fasting glucose (IFG) should be given counseling on weight loss of 5% to 10% of body weight as well as on increasing physical activity to at least 150 min/wk to prevent progression to diabetes. American Diabetes Association (ADA) recommends screening patients older than 45 years with a body mass index (BMI) greater than or equal to 25 for diabetes with fasting glucose every 3 years. Testing should be considered at a younger age or performed more frequently for those who are overweight and have 1 or more risk factors for diabetes.

Comorbidities of Obesity 271

Kavitha Bhat Schelbert

Obesity, especially visceral adiposity, is associated with morbidity and mortality through endocrine and mechanical processes. Clinical manifestations due to effects of obesity on the cardiovascular, respiratory, gastrointestinal, musculoskeletal, immune, and integumentary systems have been described. Further studies are needed to understand the pathologic processes underlying these clinical manifestations to improve disease prevention.

nutritional supplements, nutrient-limited diets, and energy-limited diets. A brief discussion of nutritional considerations relevant to other weight-loss strategies—pharmacologic, surgical, and exercise-based—is included. Specific evidence-based recommendations are presented.

Exercise and Obesity **379**

Douglas M. Okay, Paul V. Jackson, Marek Marcinkiewicz, and M. Novella Papino

Obesity and overweight are linked to a wide range of medical conditions, such as hypertension, diabetes mellitus, osteoarthritis, obstructive sleep apnea, and coronary artery disease. Overweight and obese patients who are unable to lose weight with diet alone can benefit from well-structured exercise. Potentially, an individual exercise prescription can become one of the most important components of an obesity treatment program, along with an appropriate diet. Short-term (<6 months of duration) interventions consisting of exercise combined with appropriate diet and counseling can produce a significant weight loss. No consensus exists on the amount of physical activity necessary to maintain the weight loss achieved during a short-term intervention. Long-term intervention is frequently influenced by weight regain related to complex interactions between physiologic and psychosocial factors.

Complementary and Alternative Therapies for Weight Loss **395**

Terrence E. Steyer and Adrienne Ables

Although many complementary therapies are promoted for the treatment of obesity, few are truly therapeutic. Evidence suggests that food containing diacylglycerol oil, acupuncture, and hypnosis are the only evidence-based complementary therapies for the treatment of obesity, and, at best, these should be used as adjuvants to the more conventional therapies of calorie restriction and exercise.

Pharmacotherapy for the Obese Patient **407**

Lori M. Dickerson and Peter J. Carek

The long-term safety of many antiobesity pharmacologic regimens has not been adequately evaluated. If recommended and prescribed, pharmacologic agents should be an adjunct to a structured diet and exercise regimen. Unfortunately, weight gain after discontinuation of antiobesity agents is common. In addition, the effect of weight loss obtained through the use of pharmacotherapeutic agents on overall morbidity and mortality has not been established.

Surgical Treatment of Obesity **417**

Megan K. Baker, T. Karl Byrne, and Mark E. Feldmann

Once an obese patient has failed attempts at diet modification, physical activity, pharmacologic treatment, and possibly even complementary

and alternative therapies, the next step is to consider surgical management. Treatment plans must be customized for individual patients and should involve evaluation by the primary care provider, a dietician, psychologist, and surgeon. Then depending on the individual's needs, comorbidities, and candidacy, a specific surgical intervention may be necessary. These procedures are restrictive, malabsorptive, and a combination of both. Each procedure has its own short-term and long-term complications and must be monitored for the rest of the individual's life.

FORTHCOMING ISSUES

September 2009

Cancer: What the Primary Care Practitioner Needs to Know, Part I
Richard Wender, MD, and
Danielle Snyderman, MD,
Guest Editors

December 2009

Cancer: What the Primary Care Practitioner Needs to Know, Part II
Richard Wender, MD, and
Danielle Snyderman, MD,
Guest Editors

March 2010

Integrative Medicine, Part I: Incorporating Complementary/Alternative Modalities
J. Adam Rindfleisch, MD,
Guest Editor

RECENT ISSUES

March 2009

Women's Health
Joel J. Heidelbaugh, MD,
and Wendy S. Biggs, MD,
Guest Editors

December 2008

Wellness and Prevention
Vincent Morelli, MD,
and Roger Zoorob, MD, MPH,
Guest Editors

September 2008

Kidney Diseases and Hypertension, Part II
Edgar V. Lerma, MD, FACP, FASN, FAHA,
Guest Editor

ISSUES OF RELATED INTEREST

Medical Clinics of North America, January 2009 (Vol. 93, No. 1)
Osteoarthritis
David J. Hunter, *Guest Editor*
Available at: www.medical.theclinics.com

Clinics in Geriatric Medicine, May 2008 (Vol. 24, No. 2)
Pain Management
Howard S. Smith, *Guest Editor*
Available at: www.geriatric.theclinics.com

Foreword

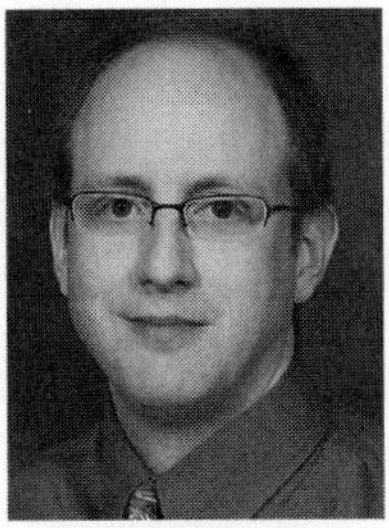

Joel J. Heidelbaugh, MD
Consulting Editor

Obesity has been labeled as "a modern-day epidemic" and everyone knows it. The lay press is riddled with countless magazine covers and articles, diets and cookbooks, and self-help books and programs. Weight loss clinics and programs are plentiful, while pills and remedies that promise results continue to increase in popularity. The obesity epidemic is costing our healthcare system billions of dollars annually and will continue to do so. The frightening point is that our society recognizes this grave issue and seems to be losing the famed "battle of the bulge," as national obesity rates continue to skyrocket. Searching for the most current and disparaging data, I googled "*obesity statistics*" and clicked on the first link, which is the Centers for Disease Control and Prevention's compilation of US Obesity Trends from 1985 to 2007.[1] This website takes you directly to 30 seconds of colorfully horrifying statistics, which highlight the increases in obesity prevalence from state to state over the last 2 decades. Further exploration of this website details gender and racial disparities in obesity, which parallel national morbidity and mortality statistics.

The harsh reality is that most of the clinicians in practice today have been inadequately trained to manage and treat obesity and to ultimately prevent its numerous complications. I am ashamed to say that I did not even have a single nutrition class in 4 years of medical school! Equally discouraging is the fact that most health insurance plans do not cover basic nutrition counseling unless a patient has significant comorbidities, and even then, it is often grossly inadequate. The greatest chance of success that we as clinicians have in preventing and treating obesity is to educate ourselves, so that we can best educate and motivate our patients. It is no longer acceptable to tell our patients that they are obese; we must tell them *how* to lose weight and support them until they reach their weight loss goals. Obesity is rivaling accidents and injuries as the leading cause of disability in the United States. Further research is desperately needed to understand the complex pathways that interplay among the endocrine, neurologic, and gastrointestinal systems so that new pharmacologic treatment options can be created, trialed, and put into everyday medical practice. New approaches to cognitive and behavioral therapy will also provide an important avenue of support.

Prim Care Clin Office Pract 36 (2009) xiii–xiv
doi:10.1016/j.pop.2009.02.002 primarycare.theclinics.com

Surgical options for obesity treatment are showing great promise in many people over the short term, and these cohorts will be closely followed for complications and post-operative weight gain.

I sincerely thank Dr. Ann Rodden and Dr.Vanessa Diaz for rising to the challenge of creating a volume of outstanding review articles dedicated to the challenging topic of obesity management. The breadth of subtopics herein, all authored by expert clinicians, renders this issue of *Primary Care* a must read for primary care clinicians as well as their residents and students. This vast amount of practical knowledge should significantly augment the care and support we deliver to our many obese patients on a daily basis. Perhaps sophisticated and motivated patients who struggle with controlling their obesity can also learn firsthand from these pages and live happier, longer, and more prosperous lives.

Joel J. Heidelbaugh, MD
Departments of Family Medicine and Urology
University of Michigan Medical School
Ann Arbor, MI

Ypsilanti Health Center
200 Arnet Suite 200
Ypsilanti, MI 48198

E-mail address:
jheidel@umich.edu (J.J. Heidelbaugh)

REFERENCE

1. US Obesity Trends 1985–2007. Available at: http://www.cdc.gov/nccdphp/dnpa/obesity/trend/maps/. Accessed February 22, 2009.

Preface

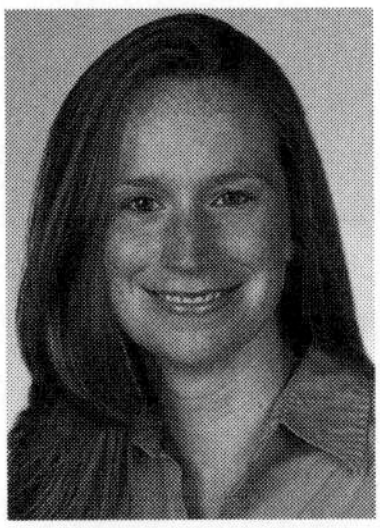
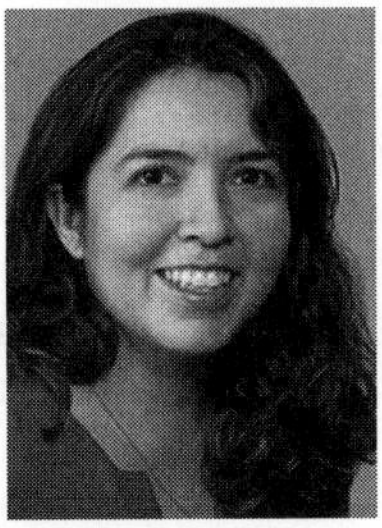

Ann Rodden, DO, MS Vanessa Diaz, MD, MS
Guest Editors

The obesity epidemic continues to plague the United States with no end in sight, leading to poor health outcomes and increased health care costs. Poor dietary choices and sedentary lifestyles are major factors that influence the development of obesity. Of course, other factors (such as genetics, medical conditions, and medications themselves) can also contribute to the problem. It is not just the mass effect from the actual weight a person has on him or her that is concerning but also the effect that weight has metabolically on every system of the body. Economic issues due to obesity have wide-ranging impact, such as airlines having to buy more gas now than in the past due to the increased weight of passengers. However, the major concern is the impact of obesity on health, causing conditions such as type 2 diabetes mellitus, hypertension, sleep apnea, and arthritis, to name just a few.

Developing an approach to addressing the obesity epidemic can be overwhelming. The lack of easy, effective solutions can be discouraging. So what can we, as primary care providers, do? Early identification of overweight and obesity is an initial key step. If people do not realize they are overweight or obese, then they may slip through the cracks and not get help until they are morbidly obese or already have comorbidities from the excess weight. Second, it is necessary to determine whether other comorbidities are present. Developing an individualized treatment plan with realistic goals is the final step, with continued monitoring over time. Counseling those who are not overweight to avoid weight gain and discussing the prevention of obesity with parents are also important.

Identification of obesity requires screening every person that comes into the office, as looks may be misleading. Screening usually consists of checking a body mass index (BMI), which is currently the standard measure of obesity. However, BMI may not be an accurate measure at the currently accepted threshold levels due to differences in body composition by race and ethnicity and changes during the aging process. Certain ethnicities may be more prone to having visceral adiposity at lower BMIs, and the

Prim Care Clin Office Pract 36 (2009) xv–xvii
doi:10.1016/j.pop.2009.02.001 **primarycare.theclinics.com**

current measures we use to determine overweight and obesity were determined in only one group: whites. Also, some cultures, such as blacks, tend not to identify themselves as overweight or obese and are accepting of higher BMIs. If an individual does not feel the need to lose weight, he or she is less likely to try.

The next step, identifying comorbidities, consists of not only determining medical conditions in general but also physical medical conditions and psychological disorders that may prevent your patient from success in weight loss. Having arthritis of the knees may prevent someone from exercising to lose weight, just as depression or binge eating may sabotage the implementation of healthy dietary changes. Thus, appropriate identification and treatment of comorbidities is relevant to improving health outcomes directly, as well as to promoting weight loss.

The last step consists of treatment of the obesity and comorbidities. Studies are currently underway to identify the most effective approaches to fighting obesity. Lifestyle changes that promote healthy nutrition and physical activity are the mainstay of any weight loss treatment and plan for ongoing maintenance of a healthy weight. But it is difficult to motivate individuals to make these lifestyle changes. Concerning children and adolescents, the American Academy of Pediatrics has developed a four-step process in the treatment of overweight and obese children. Also, motivational interviewing with parents and the child may strengthen the doctor–patient relationship and give insight into the home situation leading to the weight gain. In adults, a set recommendation for dietary changes and physical activity has not been determined, but many organizations are currently researching this. Knowledge of nutrition guidelines coupled with an accurate assessment of dietary intake is the starting point for the development of an individualized weight loss plan. A nutrition and exercise prescription to improve dietary choices and slowly integrate exercise into everyday life is one method to improve nutrition and physical activity. Such a prescription requires the patient and provider to find changes in diet and physical activities the patient would like to and is willing to do, as well as determining a schedule for the patient to implement these changes. This sets some structure and solidifies the lifestyle modification plan, rather than merely counseling that exercise is good or that the patient needs to eat better.

Other resources are also available to assist in weight loss. These include the use of complementary and alternative treatments, pharmacologic treatments, and surgical interventions. Unfortunately, data are limited on the effectiveness and safety of complementary and alternative treatments. A number of pharmacologic treatments are approved for weight loss by the United States Food and Drug Administration (FDA), but data on their long-term effectiveness are also limited. Some of these treatments may lead to a small weight loss, which for some can be a starting point to motivate further weight loss. For many, though, these modalities are short-term answers to a bigger problem, and when discontinued can lead to weight regain. The last treatment modality for weight loss is bariatric surgery. Over the years, bariatric surgery has evolved into a laproscopic procedure that can be fine-tuned to the needs of the patient. Initially, only adults had this procedure, but now adolescents are also going under the knife.

Overall, the pages to follow in this issue of *Primary Care: Clinics in Office Practice* include an evidence-based review of the relationship obesity has with the human body (physical and mental) and how we, as providers, can treat it with nutrition, physical activity, pharmacologic measures, complementary and alternative treatments, and, finally, bariatric surgery. This review also delves into the impact of obesity on special populations, such as minorities, children and adolescents, and women of childbearing age.

Ann Rodden, DO, MS
Department of Family Medicine
Medical University of South Carolina
295 Calhoun Street
Charleston, SC 29425

Vanessa Diaz, MD, MS
Department of Family Medicine
Medical University of South Carolina
295 Calhoun Street
Charleston, SC 29425

E-mail addresses:
rodden@musc.edu (A. Rodden)
diazva@musc.edu (V. Diaz)

Obesity on the Rise

Debra Boardley, PhD, RD[a,b,*], Rebecca S. Pobocik, PhD, RD[b,c]

KEYWORDS

• Obesity • Overweight • Anthropometric measures
• Epidermiology • Health care costs • Public health

Obesity is one of the greatest public health challenges in the United States. This article covers the epidemiology of obesity, anthropometric measures, and the costs of obesity to society.

EPIDEMIOLOGY

Definitions

The World Health Organization (WHO) considers obesity a disease and defines it as excess body fat to the extent that health is impaired.[1] In both adults and children, obesity is commonly assessed with the BMI calculated using weight and height (kg/m^2). The WHO currently defines adult overweight and obesity by using BMI cutoff points of 25 and 30 kg/m^2, respectively. National Heart, Lung, and Blood Institute (NHLBI) and the North American Association for the Study of Obesity Committee also recommend these cutoff points.[2] NHLBI and WHO identify subcategories: underweight less than 18.5 kg/m^2; normal weight 18.5 to 24.9 kg/m^2; overweight 25 to 29.9 kg/m^2; obesity (Class I) 30 to 34.9 kg/m^2; obesity (Class II) 35 to 39.9 kg/m^2; and extreme obesity (Class III) greater than or equal to 40 kg/m^2. Additionally, NHLBI recommends using WC cutoff points of 40 in (102 cm) for men and 35 in (88 cm) for women to define central or abdominal obesity. When used together, increased BMI and increased WC are positively associated with heart disease, hypertension, and type 2 diabetes mellitus.[2]

The definition of overweight and obesity in children and adolescents is more complex. In children, BMI changes with age during stages of growth. Previous category definitions for children used the terms "at risk of overweight" and "overweight." To address the issue of childhood obesity, an Expert Committee convened by the American Medical Association in collaboration with the Department of Health and Human Services' Health Resources and Services Administration and the Centers for

[a] Department of Public Health, College of Medicine, University of Toledo, 2801 W Bancroft Mail Stop 119, Toledo, OH 43606, USA
[b] Northwest Ohio Consortium for Public Health, Mail Stop 1042, 3000 Arlington Avenue, Toledo, OH 43614, USA
[c] Department of Nutrition, School of Family and Consumer Sciences, Bowling Green State University, 302 Johnston Hall, Bowling Green, OH 43403-0059, USA
* Corresponding author. Department of Public Health, College of Medicine, University of Toledo, 2801 W Bancroft Mail Stop 119, Toledo, OH 43606.
E-mail address: debra.boardley@utoledo.edu (D. Boardley).

Prim Care Clin Office Pract 36 (2009) 243–255
doi:10.1016/j.pop.2009.01.003 primarycare.theclinics.com
0095-4543/09/$ – see front matter

Disease Control and Prevention (CDC) recommends that children and adolescents (2–19 years) with a BMI greater than or equal to the 95th percentile for age and sex be considered obese and those with BMI greater than or equal to the 85th percentile and less than the 95th percentile for age and sex be considered overweight.[3]

In Children and Adolescents

Among children aged 6 to 19 years, 31% exceed the 85th percentile, and 16% exceed the 95th percentile (now classified obese).[4] Increases in BMI with time vary for different age and racial groups.[5] The prevalence of obesity in children increased from 1971 to 1974 and 1999 to 2000 about 4-fold, with the largest increase among 12- to 17-year-old African American adolescents, according to the National Health and Nutrition Examination Survey (NHANES). Minority children overall have higher rates of obesity than those of Caucasian children.[4–15] By race, 31% of Hispanic, 23% of African American, 16% of Caucasian, and 14% of Asian children are obese.[5,13] Preschools in Chicago that have predominantly Caucasian children have 24% of children more than normal weight, whereas centers with predominantly African American children have 39.5%, and those with predominantly Hispanic children have 40.2%.[16] The Healthy Kids Project has similar results to those of other studies with school-aged children: 30.8% of students are overweight and 28.5% obese.[17]

Socioeconomic status (SES) relates to rates of overweight and obesity for some children and adolescents. In families below the poverty line, older adolescents (15–17 years) are more likely to be overweight, but no effect is seen on younger adolescents (12–14 years).[18] The relationship of childhood overweight and family income varies by race.[19] For Hispanic children, lower family income is related to increasing BMI percentile. Among African American children, increased family income is associated with increased BMI, and among Caucasian children, prevalence of overweight is fairly constant.[20] As the rates of obesity in children increase, SES inequalities are diminishing with time.[21] With the large increases in obesity, both low- and high-SES groups may be affected.

Persistence of childhood overweight into adulthood affects the prevalence of adult obesity.[22] Most obese adolescents (ages 13–20 years) in the National Longitudinal Study of Adolescent Health remain obese as they become adults (ages 19–26 years).[23] Approximately 85% of obese adolescents are obese adults. Among overweight children, 65% of Caucasian girls and 84% of African American girls become obese adults, whereas 71% of Caucasian boys and 82% of African American boys remain obese.[24] Interestingly, thin Caucasian boys (BMI $\leq$ the 50th percentile) tend to gain more weight in adulthood than their African American counterparts and have a higher prevalence of overweight.

In Adults

The most recent NHANES data (1999-2004) estimate that among adult men and women (20 years or older), 66.3% are overweight or obese, 32.4% are obese, and 4.8% are extremely obese.[25,26] Currently, the lifetime risk of being overweight is estimated to exceed 70% and that for obesity exceeds 35%.[27] The prevalence of overweight and obese adults has increased from 1,950 to 2,000 for both men and women, with the largest increase in BMI greater than 35.[28,29]

As obesity rises, so does the WC and abdominal obesity. For men, the prevalence of abdominal obesity changed from 12.7% in 1960 to 1962 to 29% in 1988 to 1994 and later 38.3% in 1999 to 2000.[30] For women during the same time periods, the prevalence of abdominal obesity increased from 19.4% to 38.8% and then 59.9%.

Abdominal obesity has increased in both sexes in African Americans and Caucasians; but in Hispanics, the increase has been seen only in men.[31]

Similar to children, gender, age, race, and SES all influence the prevalence of adult obesity.[32–35] In the United States, men are more likely to be overweight than women; however, women are more likely to be obese.[4] The prevalence of overweight increases with age, with more than 70% of persons 60 years or older being overweight or obese.[4,26] The burden of obesity is higher in minority groups when compared with that in Caucasians in the United States, with 64.2% of Caucasians, 76.1% of African Americans, and 75.8% of Hispanics being overweight or obese.[25,26,33] Racial disparities are greatest for women, as 58.0% of Caucasian women are overweight or obese compared with 81.6% of African American women and 75.4% of Hispanic women.[4,16,25]

The rate of obesity greatly increased in the years between 1971 and 2000, whereas the disparity in obesity rates across SES decreased.[34] SES factors have a stronger impact in Caucasians than in minority groups, with a negative association between SES and obesity in Caucasian men and women but a positive association in African American men and Hispanic men.[35] African American women, however, who grew up in the most disadvantaged households have obesity levels more than twice as high as those of women from less impoverished backgrounds.[36] For minority women, in addition to low individual SES (income, education, assets), living in a socioeconomically disadvantaged community increases the prevalence of obesity.[32]

In addition to SES, education level and choice of occupation have associations with obesity for some race and gender. A 4-year cohort of middle-aged women found that African American women and Caucasian women have similar BMI at the lowest level of education (high school or less).[37] The BMI of African American women is higher than that of Caucasian women at the moderate (some college) and highest (college degree or more) levels of education. Compared with Caucasian college students, African Americans and Hispanics are more likely to be overweight, whereas Asian students are less likely to be so. When comparing by gender, male college students are more likely to be overweight and obese than their female counterparts.[38]

Occupation may be a variable in obesity according to the National Health Interview Survey.[39] Workers in 41 occupation categories participated and identified African American female workers as having the highest prevalence of obesity. For male workers, vehicle operators (31.7%), police, and firefighters (29.8%) have the highest rates of obesity, with no occupational groups having obesity rates less than 11% for men. For women, vehicle operators (31.0%) and protective service workers (30.5%) have the highest rates of obesity, whereas architects and surveyors (7.3%) and construction and extractive trade workers (6.9%) have the lowest rates.[39]

ANTHROPOMETRIC MEASURES

Obesity can be assessed by direct and indirect methods. Indirect methods are most suitable for clinical and field applications, because they do not require expensive equipment and are easily implemented.[40] Anthropometric measures include BMI, WC, waist-to-height ratio (W/Ht), waist-to-hip ratio (WHR), and sagittal trunk diameter.

Adults

Body mass index

BMI, an estimate of body fat percentage, is currently the standard indirect measure of obesity and overweight.[40,41] BMI works as well as densitometry for the estimation of overweight and metabolic risk.[42,43] Thus, at the population level, BMI is an adequate index of obesity-related metabolic risk. Limitations to BMI are that it does not distinguish between fat mass and lean mass; the cutoff values may be different in the elderly and non-Caucasian populations; and it does not capture body fat distribution, such as increased abdominal fat accumulation.[40,41]

Different BMI cutoff points have been proposed for specific ethnic populations. Chinese, Malay, Indian, Taiwanese, and Indonesian men and women have more body fat than do Caucasians for a given BMI, due, in part, to different body proportions, which means that Asian people are at risk for chronic disease at BMIs lower than the existing cutoff point for overweight.[2,40,44] Thus, additional BMI cutoff points are suggested with Asian populations.[44] In some groups of Asians, a BMI of 23 rather than 25 would indicate increased risk from overweight and a BMI of 27.5 rather than 30 would indicate increased risk from obesity.[44]

Waist circumference

Unlike the BMI, WC is a means of identifying abdominal obesity, which is associated with visceral adipose tissue mass.[2,41,45] Central adiposity is highly correlated with hypertension, coronary heart disease, type 2 diabetes mellitus, and increased mortality risk. The cutoff points of 102 cm for men and 88 cm for women, originally based on regression curves that identified the WC values associated with BMI classifications of overweight ($\geq$25 kg/m^2), are most appropriate for Caucasian adults.[40,46]

WC is complicated by the heterogeneity of measurement sites and techniques.[41,42,47–51] Some authorities suggest the midpoint between the lowest rib and the iliac crest, while others suggest immediately above the iliac crest.[42] WC measurements are not comparable at 4 of the most commonly used sites and are, thus, not interchangeable; however, there is no uniformly accepted approach.[52] Each WC site correlates with trunk fat and total body fat for both sexes. For the clinical evaluation of overweight, the NHLBI expert panel recommends measuring the horizontal plane around the abdomen at the level of the iliac crest, and the consensus panel Shaping America's Health recommends placing a nonstretchable tape "around the patient's bare midriff, after the patient exhales while standing without shoes and with both feet touching and arms hanging freely."[2,45] The tape should be placed perpendicular to the long axis of the body and horizontal to the floor with sufficient tension to conform to the body.[45]

Asian ethnic groups generally have more visceral fat at smaller WCs than that of Caucasians, suggesting lower WC cutoff points for these populations.[40] A study of 2,050 subjects proposes WC cutoffs values for adult Asian Indians of 78 cm for men and 72 cm for women.[48] A WC cutoff of 90 cm for men and 80 cm for women identifies higher cardiovascular risk and a BMI level of 25. The WHO is currently investigating ethnicity-specific WC cutoff points.[44]

The combination of BMI and WC is especially good for assessing obesity and evaluating risk for diabetes and cardiovascular disease.[2,40,49,51] BMI and WC should be used together in clinical settings.[2]

Waist-to-height ratio

Some researchers recommend that the W/Ht ratio and WC (in inches) divided by the height (in inches) should be used as the global indicator for health risk of obesity, because it is a simple, inexpensive measurement; it is associated with risk factors for obesity and metabolic syndrome; and it works equally well for both men and women, people in different ethnic groups, and for children and adults.[53] This index can identify people within the normal range of BMI who may have a higher metabolic risk associated with central obesity. A boundary value of 0.5 is used to keep WC less than half of height.[53]

To assess the value of anthropometric measures, researchers measure a large number of people using direct assessment methods (ie, dual-energy X-ray absorptiometry) and develop optimal indexes and equations for predicting absolute body fat and percentage body fat. The theoretical indexes and equations are then tested in a separate group of individuals to determine which index or equation best predicts actual body fat (absolute or percentage) or metabolic condition. One such study found that W/Ht is the best predictor of absolute body fat, whereas BMI is the best predictor of body fat percentage, suggesting that W/Ht may be a more optimal index than BMI, particularly at high body weights.[47] Additionally, W/Ht has the highest correlation with percent fat mass, is the best predictor of risk in patients with metabolic syndrome, and is equal to BMI in predicting diabetes.[42,43] More research is needed before this measure is accepted as the national standard.

Waist-to-hip ratio

A WHR greater than 0.8 in women and greater than 0.9 in men is a predictor of increased risk of obesity complications.[50] The WHR includes both subcutaneous and intra-abdominal adipose tissue, and it is unknown how to correct for the level of subcutaneous tissue. The WHR can be affected by postprandial status, standing position, time of day, and depth of inspiration, although the degree to which these factors can contribute to error is unknown.[50] As with WC, there is no standardized approach for measurement. In addition to the different locations for the waist measurement, the hip measurement can vary as well, but the widest area around the hips is commonly used.[41,47–49] Another practical difficulty is the more invasive nature of the hip measurement. Thus, the BMI in combination with WC is a better measure of obesity than WHR.

Sagittal trunk diameter

Sagittal trunk diameter is a less commonly used method of assessing abdominal fat. The sagittal trunk diameter is taken while subjects are in a recumbent position on an examination table and is the maximum diameter of the abdomen in the sagittal plane.[41,47] In a group of Caucasian and Asian males, the sagittal diameter most effectively identifies men with metabolic syndrome with a cutoff point of just about 27 cm, with 82.2% sensitivity and 90% specificity.[41] When a person with an enlarged intra-abdominal adipose mass is standing, gravity pulls the fat tissue down so the WC might not be as accurate in assessing the intra-abdominal fat in those who are very obese compared with when the same person lies supine and the mass shifts causing anterior projection of the abdomen, which is measured by the sagittal diameter.[41] Clinical judgment should be used in deciding if this method would produce better results than a WC measurement.

Older Adults

With aging, body composition changes and height decreases, affecting the interpretation of anthropometric data. On average, older persons have more fat than do younger adults at any given BMI.[40] When comparing noninvasive body fat estimates to percent body fat in the elderly, a reasonably high correlation exists with BMI (0.73–0.93) and with WC (0.64–0.78) to body fat percentage.[54] However, the diagnosis of obesity is less likely to be overestimated if BMI measurements are based on height measured in early life. Furthermore, absolute levels of WC indicate more visceral fat in older persons than in younger persons, because relatively more fat accumulates in the abdomen and less fat at the extremities as people age.[40] In general, BMI is a good method to diagnose obesity in older adults;[40,54] however, in those older than 70 years, sagittal trunk diameter may be a better indicator of visceral fat than either WC or BMI.[40]

Children

The CDC 2000 BMI-for-age percentiles are recommended for use with all US children regardless of ethnicity.[55,56] BMI levels used to identify overweight and obese children are used relative to age, because the upper percentiles of BMI increase dramatically with age. The BMI percentiles also must be gender specific because of the systematic physiologic differences between boys and girls.[56] The Institute of Medicine and the Expert Committee on Assessment of Child and Adolescent Overweight and Obesity recommend that individuals 2 to 18 years with BMI greater than or equal to 30 kg/m2 or greater than or equal to the 95th percentile for age and gender on the CDC 2000 growth charts should be considered obese.[57,58] This is a stronger statement than the previously recognized "overweight" because of the nature of the current epidemic and the need for medical professionals and others to address the problem actively.[56] The Expert Committee also recommends that children and adolescents with a BMI greater than or equal to the 85th percentile but less than the 95th percentile or 30 kg/m^2 now be considered overweight rather than "at risk of overweight" to emphasize the need for action.[58] For children younger than 2 years, BMI normative values are not available. For this reason, the weight-for-recumbent-length percentiles from the CDC 2000 growth charts are appropriate to use for evaluating weight relative to linear growth. Weight-for-length percentiles greater than or equal to the 95th percentile identify these children as overweight, but the term "obese" should not be used for children younger than 2 years.[56,58]

A limitation to the use of BMI for children is the potential for misclassification due to inconsistent methods and equipment. Some general practitioners have no formal training on assessing pediatric height and weight, and servicing of anthropometric equipment may occur on rare occasions.[59] Nondigital scales are less accurate than digital scales, and if a scale is placed on a soft surface, accuracy decreases even more. The most accurate height measures are obtained with stadiometers that are calibrated at regular intervals. The BMI of a 9-year-old girl may range from the 10th to the 80th percentile for age when calculated using the variability in height and weight due to equipment error when her true BMI is actually near the 50th percentile.[59]

THE COSTS TO SOCIETY

Obesity has great impact on health, particularly increasing the prevalence of obesity-related diseases including type 2 diabetes mellitus, cardiovascular disease, cancer, musculoskeletal disorders, sleep apnea, and gall bladder disease.[60] In addition to the impact on health, there is an economic cost to the consumer, government, and employers.

Cost to Individuals

The impact of obesity on mortality is a subject of controversy, with studies reporting higher rates of mortality and others reporting no impact.[61–64] The effect on life expectancy differs with age, sex, and BMI category.[61] Obesity in African Americans results in a smaller increase in mortality compared with that in Caucasians. Considering a 20-year-old with a BMI greater than or equal to 45, the Caucasian male is estimated to have 13 years' life lost due to obesity. Considering that he would be expected to live another 58 years, this represents a 22% reduction in remaining years of life.[61] A Caucasian female of same age and BMI has an 8-year or 13% reduction in remaining years of life, whereas an African American male loses 11 years (16% reduction in remaining life), and an African American female loses 5 years (9% reduction in remaining years).

Just as important as quantity, obesity can also affect quality of life. Obese adults have lower health status (measured by Medical Outcomes Study Short-Form 36-item questionnaire) and higher Beck Depression Inventory scores.[65] Overweight and obese adults are also more likely to sustain injuries that require medical treatment. The odds of sustaining a medically treated injury are 15% higher for overweight adults and 48% higher for extremely obese adults.[66] Medical conditions ranging from heart disease, diabetes, and cancer to knee replacement surgery, depression, fatigue, and insomnia are all more common in obese patients.[67]

Older adults with BMI greater than 35 are more than twice as likely as people of normal weight to report fair/poor health and twice as many chronic medical conditions.[68] Moderate obesity (BMI 30-34.9) is associated with a 50% increase in the likelihood of activities of daily life (ADL) limitation, and severe obesity has a 300% increase.[69] In older adults, obesity is associated with a 2-fold increase in the odds of ADL limitations and a reduction in ADL limitation-free years of 5.7 years for men and 5.02 years for women.[70] Obese 70-year-olds live about as long as normal-weight peers but spend more then $39,000 more on health care during their lifetime and have fewer disability-free years.[62]

Annual Medical Costs

Obese adults incur annual medical expenditures that are 36% to 37.4% higher than those of normal-weight adults.[68,71] Between 5% and 7% of annual health care expenditures can be attributed to obesity.[71] State-level costs for obesity-attributable medical expenditures are reported with a wide range from $87 million in Wyoming to $7.7 billion in California.[72] Weight-related expenditure rates are similar for men and women but vary by race.[73] Increases in BMI are associated with increases in medical expenditures in Caucasian adults, although among Hispanics and particularly African Americans BMI is not related to health care costs. The reasons for the racial discrepancies are unclear. They may be due to the observation that BMI has different effects among whites and blacks, or it may be a result of the documented disparities in care between white and minority populations.[61,73] The increase in medical expenditure costs is from more office visits for comorbid conditions, inpatient and outpatient hospital care, and prescription drugs.[71,73]

Overall, a BMI of 30 to 35 increases health care expenditures about 25%, a BMI of 35 to 40 increases them 50%, and a BMI greater than 40 doubles health care expenditures compared with those of a normal BMI group.[73–75] When considering the degree of obesity, adults with extreme or morbid obesity (BMI $\geq$ 40 kg/m^2) have health care expenditures that are 81% greater than those of normal-weight adults, 65% greater than those of overweight adults, and 47% greater than those of adults with class I obesity.[75] Increases in spending for obese patients account for more than 38% of the diabetes spending growth and 41% of heart disease spending growth.[76]

Cost to Taxpayer

Increased obesity costs are partially financed by taxpayers, primarily through Medicare and Medicaid. Half of the costs in the United States attributable to overweight and obesity are paid by Medicare and Medicaid.[71] Older obese adults are eventually covered by Medicare, which spends about 34% more on an obese recipient than that on one of normal weight.[62] The Medicaid population has a 50% higher prevalence of obesity, and as a result, the average taxpayer spends approximately $175/y to finance obesity-related medical costs among Medicare and Medicaid recipients.[71]

BMI at young and middle adulthood is significantly and positively associated with Medicare health care charges in older age.[77] For those who are overweight or obese at 65 years, men will increase lifetime health expenditures by 6% to 13%, whereas women increase them by 11% to 17%.[78] A study of military retirees found that 80% of men and 60% of women are overweight or obese and are likely to have obesity-related diseases.[79]

Costs to Business and Industry

Overweight workers increase costs to employers due to higher health care expenditures and increased absenteeism due to poor health.[80–82] BMI classification predicts high health care cost and high absence. When comparing across the 6 NHLBI groups, those in the normal-weight group have the lowest medical costs, and the medical costs increase with higher BMIs. This relationship is consistent for both males and females and also across all age groups except for the 75 years and older age group, in whom the relationship is inconsistent.[80]

About 30% of the total medical expenditures attributable to obesity are from increased absenteeism. Workers with BMI greater than 30 were 61% more likely to miss work time than workers of normal BMI. Interestingly, although only about 3% of workers have grade III obesity, they account for 21% of the obesity-related costs of absenteeism, which totaled $4.3 billion in 2004.[83]

When comparing workman's compensation claims, rates of the normal-weight employee claims are only half of the claims of the extremely obese workers. Additionally, the number of lost workdays is 13 times higher, and the cost of medical claims is 7 times higher among the heaviest employees compared with those of employees of normal weight. Much higher rates of claims are also observed in the more physically demanding jobs.[84]

The US Federal Aviation Administration (FAA) has determined that the airline industry is facing increased fuel costs due to obesity. The FAA estimates that airlines had to purchase an additional 350 million gallons of fuel in 2000 for the increase in weight of passengers.[85]

Costs for Children

Overweight children, compared with normal-weight children, have significantly higher prevalence of dyslipidemia, fasting blood glucose levels, glycohemoglobin levels, and systolic blood pressure.[86] One study found that medical expenditures are not greater for overweight children compared with those for normal-weight children and hypothesized that this finding was likely due to the greater prevalence of poverty and minority status among overweight children.[86] Other studies, however, do report that overweight children have significantly more medical visits and also use more mental health resources.[87] Another study found that laboratory use and total health care expenditures are significantly higher in children diagnosed with obesity.[88]

Similar to findings in children, adolescents with higher BMI have significantly worse self-reported health and are more likely to report a functional limitation.[89]

SUMMARY

The prevalence of obesity has increased markedly over recent years. The burden of obesity is higher in minority groups, and obesity rates vary according to SES, age, and employment. BMI and WC are the primary anthropometric measures of obesity, but weight-for-height is increasingly being found as a measure that identifies both overweight and metabolic risk. BMI should be interpreted with caution in the elderly, children, and some Asian populations. The costs of obesity to society are staggering, with effects on lifespan and quality of life, increased medical expenditures, and an increased financial burden to taxpayers, business, and industry.

REFERENCES

1. World Health Organization. Obesity: preventing and managing the global epidemic. Report of a WHO consultation. Technical report series no. 894. Geneva (Switzerland): World Health Organization; 2000.
2. National Heart, Lung, and Blood Institute. Clinical guidelines on the identification, evaluation, and treatment of overweight and obesity in adults. Bethesda (MD): National Heart, Lung, and Blood Institute; 1998.
3. American Medical Association. Expert committee recommendations on the assessment, prevention, and treatment of childhood and adolescent overweight and obesity. Chicago: American Medical Association; 2007.
4. Hedley AA, Ogden CL, Johnson CL, et al. Prevalence of overweight and obesity among US children, adolescents, and adults, 1999–2002. JAMA 2004;291(23): 2847–50.
5. Freedman DS, Khan LK, Serdula MK, et al. Racial and ethnic differences in secular trends for childhood BMI, weight, and height. Obesity 2006;14(2):301–8.
6. Gordon-Larsen P, Adair LS, Popkin BM. The relationship of ethnicity, socioeconomic factors, and overweight in US adolescents. Obes Res 2003;11(1):121–9.
7. Whitaker RC, Orzol SM. Obesity among US urban preschool children: relationships to race, ethnicity, and socioeconomic status. Arch Pediatr Adolesc Med 2006;160(6):578–84.
8. Nelson JA, Chiasson MA, Ford V. Childhood overweight in a New York City WIC population. Am J Public Health 2004;94(3):458–62.
9. Mirza NM, Kadow K, Palmer M, et al. Prevalence of overweight among inner city Hispanic-American children and adolescents. Obes Res 2004;12(8):1298–310.
10. Baruffi G, Hardy CJ, Waslien CI, et al. Ethnic differences in the prevalence of overweight among young children in Hawaii. J Am Diet Assoc 2004;104(11): 1701–7.
11. Eichner JE, Moore WE, Perveen G, et al. Overweight and obesity in an ethnically diverse rural school district: the Healthy Kids Project. Obesity (Silver Spring) 2008;16(2):501–4.
12. Wang Y, Liang H, Tussing L, et al. Obesity and related risk factors among low socio-economic status minority students in Chicago. Public Health Nutr 2007;10(9): 927–38.
13. Haas JS, Lee LB, Kaplan CP, et al. The association of race, socioeconomic status, and health insurance status with the prevalence of overweight among children and adolescents. Am J Public Health 2003;93(12):2105–10.
14. Braunschweig CL, Gomez S, Liang H, et al. Obesity and risk factors for the metabolic syndrome among low-income, urban, African American schoolchildren: the rule rather than the exception? Am J Clin Nutr 2005;81(5):970–5.
15. Patrick K, Norman GJ, Calfas KJ, et al. Diet, physical activity, and sedentary behaviors as risk factors for overweight in adolescence. Arch Pediatr Adolesc Med 2004;158(4):385–90.

16. Turner L, Hagin S. Overweight among Chicago preschool children. Public Health 2007;121(1):51–3.
17. Moore WE, Stephens A, Wilson T, et al. Body mass index and blood pressure screening in a rural public school system: the Healthy Kids Project. Prev Chronic Dis 2006;3(4):A114. Available at: http://www.cdc.gov/pcd/issues/2006/oct/05_0236.htm.
18. Miech RA, et al. Trends in the association of poverty with overweight among US adolescents, 1971–2004. JAMA 2006;295(20):2385–93.
19. Freedman DS, et al. Childhood overweight and family income. MedGenMed 2007;9(2):26.
20. Wang Y, Zhang Q. Are American children and adolescents of low socioeconomic status at increased risk of obesity? Changes in the association between overweight and family income between 1971 and 2002. Am J Clin Nutr 2006;84(4):707–16.
21. Zhang Q, Wang Y. Using concentration index to study changes in socio-economic inequality of overweight among US adolescents between 1971 and 2002. Int J Epidemiol 2007;36(4):916–25.
22. Freedman DS, et al. The relation of childhood BMI to adult adiposity: the Bogalusa Heart Study. Pediatrics 2005;115(1):22–7.
23. Gordon-Larsen P, et al. Five-year obesity incidence in the transition period between adolescence and adulthood: the National Longitudinal Study of Adolescent Health. Am J Clin Nutr 2004;80(3):569–75.
24. Freedman DS, et al. Racial differences in the tracking of childhood BMI to adulthood. Obes Res 2005;13(5):928–35.
25. Ogden CL, Carroll MD, Curtin LR, et al. Prevalence of overweight and obesity in the United States, 1999–2004. JAMA 2006;295(13):1549–55.
26. Wang Y, Beydoun MA. The obesity epidemic in the United States–gender, age, socioeconomic, racial/ethnic, and geographic characteristics: a systematic review and meta-regression analysis. Epidemiol Rev 2007;29:6–28.
27. Vasan RS, Pencina MJ, Cobain M, et al. Estimated risks for developing obesity in the Framingham Heart Study. Ann Intern Med 2005;143(7):473–80.
28. Flegal KM. Epidemiologic aspects of overweight and obesity in the United States. Physiol Behav 2005;86(5):599–602.
29. Parikh NI, Pencina MJ, Wang TJ, et al. Increasing trends in incidence of overweight and obesity over 5 decades. Am J Med 2007;120(3):242–50.
30. Okosun IS, Chandra KM, Boev A, et al. Abdominal adiposity in U.S. adults: prevalence and trends, 1960–2000. Prev Med 2004;39(1):197–206.
31. Okosun IS, Choi ST, Boltri JM, et al. Trends of abdominal adiposity in white, black, and Mexican-American adults, 1988 to 2000. Obes Res 2003;11(8):1010–7.
32. Robert SA, Reither EN. A multilevel analysis of race, community disadvantage, and body mass index among adults in the US. Soc Sci Med 2004;59(12):2421–34.
33. Flegal KM, Ogden CL, Carroll MD. Prevalence and trends in overweight in Mexican-American adults and children. Nutr Rev 2004;62(7 Pt 2):S144–8.
34. Zhang Q, Wang Y. Trends in the association between obesity and socioeconomic status in U.S. adults: 1971 to 2000. Obes Res 2004;12(10):1622–32.
35. Zhang Q, Wang Y. Socioeconomic inequality of obesity in the United States: do gender, age, and ethnicity matter? Soc Sci Med 2004;58(6):1171–80.
36. James SA, Fowler-Brown A, Raghunathan TE, et al. Life-course socioeconomic position and obesity in African American Women: the Pitt County Study. Am J Public Health 2006;96(3):554–60.
37. Lewis TT, Everson-Rose, Sternfeld B, et al. Race, education, and weight change in a biracial sample of women at midlife. Arch Intern Med 2005;165(5):545–51.

38. Nelson TF, Gortmaker SL, Subramanian SV, et al. Disparities in overweight and obesity among US college students. Am J Health Behav 2007;31(4):363–73.
39. Caban AJ, et al. Obesity in US workers: The National Health Interview Survey, 1986 to 2002. Am J Public Health 2005;95(9):1614–22.
40. Snijder MB, et al. What aspects of body fat are particularly hazardous and how do we measure them? Int J Epidemiol 2006;35(1):83–92.
41. Valsamakis G, et al. Association of simple anthropometric measures of obesity with visceral fat and the metabolic syndrome in male Caucasian and Indo-Asian subjects. Diabet Med 2004;21(12):1339–45.
42. Bosy-Westphal A, et al. Value of body fat mass vs anthropometric obesity indices in the assessment of metabolic risk factors. Int J Obes (Lond) 2006;30(3):475–83.
43. Tulloch-Reid MK, et al. Do measures of body fat distribution provide information on the risk of type 2 diabetes in addition to measures of general obesity? Comparison of anthropometric predictors of type 2 diabetes in Pima Indians. Diabetes Care 2003;26(9):2556–61.
44. World Health Organization. World Health Organization Global Database on Body Mass Index. Geneva (Switzerland): World Health Organization; 2006.
45. Klein S, et al. Waist circumference and cardiometabolic risk: a consensus statement from Shaping America's Health: Association for Weight Management and Obesity Prevention; NAASO, The Obesity Society; the American Society for Nutrition; and the American Diabetes Association. Am J Clin Nutr 2007;85(5):1197–202.
46. Lean M, Han T, Morrison CE. Waist circumference as a measure for indicating need for weight management. BMJ 1995;311(6998):158–61.
47. Larsson I, et al. Optimized predictions of absolute and relative amounts of body fat from weight, height, other anthropometric predictors, and age 1. Am J Clin Nutr 2006;83(2):252–9.
48. Misra A, et al. Waist circumference cutoff points and action levels for Asian Indians for identification of abdominal obesity. Int J Obes (Lond) 2006;30(1):106–11.
49. Mamtani MR, Kulkarni HR. Predictive performance of anthropometric indexes of central obesity for the risk of type 2 diabetes. Arch Med Res 2005;36(5):581–9.
50. Moyad MA. Fad diets and obesity—Part I: measuring weight in a clinical setting. Urol Nurs 2004;24(2):114–9.
51. dos Santos RE, et al. Relationship of body fat distribution by waist circumference, dual-energy X-ray absorptiometry and ultrasonography to insulin resistance by homeostasis model assessment and lipid profile in obese and non-obese postmenopausal women. Gynecol Endocrinol 2005;21(5):295–301.
52. Wang J, et al. Comparisons of waist circumferences measured at 4 sites. Am J Clin Nutr 2003;77(2):379–84.
53. Ashwell M, Hsieh SD. Six reasons why the waist-to-height ratio is a rapid and effective global indicator for health risks of obesity and how its use could simplify the international public health message on obesity. Int J Food Sci Nutr 2005;56(5):303–7.
54. McTigue KM, Hess R, Ziouras J. Obesity in older adults: a systematic review of the evidence for diagnosis and treatment. Obesity (Silver Spring) 2006;14(9):1485–97.
55. Freedman DS, et al. Relation of BMI to fat and fat-free mass among children and adolescents. Int J Obes (Lond) 2005;29(1):1–8.
56. Krebs N, Himes J, Jacobson D, et al. Assessment of child and adolescent overweight and obesity. Pediatrics 2007;120(Suppl 4):S193–228.

57. Koplan JP, Liverman CT, Kraak VI, editors. Preventing childhood obesity: health in the balance. Washington, DC: National Academies Press; 2005.
58. Barlow S, Barlow SE. Expert committee recommendations regarding the prevention, assessment, and treatment of child and adolescent overweight and obesity: summary report. Pediatrics 2007;120(Suppl 4):S164–92.
59. Gerner B, et al. Are general practitioners equipped to detect child overweight/obesity? Survey and audit. J Paediatr Child Health 2006;42(4):206–11.
60. Stein CJ, Colditz GA. The epidemic of obesity. J Clin Endocrinol Metab 2004; 89(6):2522–5.
61. Fontaine KR, et al. Years of life lost due to obesity. JAMA 2003;289(2):187–93.
62. Lakdawalla DN, Goldman DP, Shang B. The health and cost consequences of obesity among the future elderly. Health Aff 2005;24(Suppl 2):W5R30–41.
63. Reynolds SL, Saito Y, Crimmins EM. The impact of obesity on active life expectancy in older American men and women. Gerontologist 2005;45(4):438–44.
64. Peeters A, et al. Obesity in adulthood and its consequences for life expectancy: a life-table analysis. Ann Intern Med 2003;138(1):24–32.
65. Bertakis KD, Azari R. Obesity and the use of health care services. Obes Res 2005;13(2):372–9.
66. Finkelstein EA, et al. The relationship between obesity and injuries among U.S. adults. Am J Health Promot 2007;21(5):460–8.
67. Patterson RE, et al. A comprehensive examination of health conditions associated with obesity in older adults. Am J Prev Med 2004;27(5):385–90.
68. Sturm R, Ringel JS, Andreyeva T. Increasing obesity rates and disability trends. Health Aff 2004;23(2):199–205.
69. Wolf AM, et al. Effects of lifestyle intervention on health care costs: Improving Control with Activity and Nutrition (ICAN). J Am Diet Assoc 2007;107(8): 1365–73.
70. Peeters A, et al. Adult obesity and the burden of disability throughout life. Obes Res 2004;12(7):1145–51.
71. Finkelstein EA, Fiebelkorn IC, Wang G. National medical spending attributable to overweight and obesity: how much, and who's paying? Health Affairs 2003;W3-219–26.
72. Finkelstein EA, Fiebelkorn IC, Wang G. State-level estimates of annual medical expenditures attributable to obesity. Obes Res 2004;12(1):18–24.
73. Wee CC, et al. Health care expenditures associated with overweight and obesity among US adults: importance of age and race. Am J Public Health 2005;95(1): 159–65.
74. Andreyeva T, Sturm R, Ringel JS. Moderate and severe obesity have large differences in health care costs. Obes Res 2004;12(12):1936–43.
75. Arterburn DE, Maciejewski ML, Tsevat J. Impact of morbid obesity on medical expenditures in adults. Int J Obes 2005;29(3):334–9.
76. Thorpe KE, et al. The impact of obesity on rising medical spending. Health Affairs 2004;W4-480–6.
77. Daviglus ML, et al. Relation of body mass index in young adulthood and middle age to Medicare expenditures in older age. JAMA 2004;292(22):2743–9.
78. Yang Z, Hall AG. The financial burden of overweight and obesity among elderly Americans: the dynamics of weight, longevity, and health care cost. Health Serv Res 2008;43(3):849–68.
79. Kress AM, Hartzel MC, Peterson MR. Burden of disease associated with overweight and obesity among U.S. military retirees and their dependents, aged 38–64, 2003. Prev Med 2005;41(1):63–9.

80. Bungum T, et al. The relationship of body mass index, medical costs, and job absenteeism. Am J Health Behav 2003;27(4):456–62.
81. Wang F, et al. The relationship between National Heart, Lung, and Blood Institute Weight Guidelines and concurrent medical costs in a manufacturing population. Am J Health Promot 2003;17(3):183–9.
82. Finkelstein E, Fiebelkorn C, Wang G. The costs of obesity among full-time employees. Am J Health Promot 2005;20(1):45–51.
83. Cawley J, Rizzo JA, Haas K. Occupation-specific absenteeism costs associated with obesity and morbid obesity. J Occup Environ Med 2007;49(12):1317–24.
84. Ostbye T, Dement JM, Krause KM. Obesity and workers' compensation: results from the Duke Health and Safety Surveillance System. Arch Intern Med 2007; 167(8):766–73.
85. Dannenberg AL, Burton DC, Jackson RJ. Economic and environmental costs of obesity: the impact on airlines. Am J Prev Med 2004;27(3):264.
86. Skinner AC, et al. Health status and health care expenditures in a nationally representative sample: how do overweight and healthy-weight children compare? Pediatrics 2008;121(2):269–77.
87. Estabrooks PA, Shetterly S. The prevalence and health care use of overweight children in an integrated health care system. Arch Pediatr Adolesc Med 2007; 161(3):222–7.
88. Hampl SE, et al. Resource utilization and expenditures for overweight and obese children. Arch Pediatr Adolesc Med 2007;161(1):11–4.
89. Swallen KC, et al. Overweight, obesity, and health-related quality of life among adolescents: the National Longitudinal Study of Adolescent Health. Pediatrics 2005;115(2):340–7.

Obesity and Metabolic Disease

Richelle J. Koopman, MD, MS[a,*], Sarah J. Swofford, MD[a], Mark N. Beard, MD[a,b], Susan E. Meadows, MLS[a,c]

KEYWORDS

- Obesity • Diabetes mellitus • Cardiovascular disease
- Metabolic syndrome • Polycystic ovary syndrome
- Insulin resistance

OBESITY AND DIABETES

Epidemiology

The estimated prevalence of diabetes among US adults in 2002 was 9.3%.[1] This is expected to rise to 14.5% by 2031.[2] The risk of developing type 2 diabetes increases with age, obesity, lack of exercise, poor diet, and smoking.[3] Other risk factors include family history of diabetes, race/ethnicity (African Americans, Latinos, Native Americans, Asian-Americans, and Pacific Islanders), previously identified IFG or IGT, history of gestational diabetes, hypertension (HTN), low levels of high-density lipoprotein (HDL) and/or elevated levels of triglycerides, polycystic ovary syndrome (PCOS), and history of cardiovascular disease (CVD).[4] About 85% of all US adults with diabetes are overweight or obese.[5] Although both physical inactivity and obesity are significant predictors of developing diabetes, obesity is the strongest independent risk factor for diabetes.[6] Compared with women who are normal weight, the relative risk for diabetes associated with obesity ranges from 9.9 to 20.1.[3,6,7] The risk of diabetes in men who are obese is about 8 times higher than that of those who are not obese (RR 7.9–8.3).[7,8]

Pathophysiology

Although obesity is a major risk factor for development of type 2 diabetes, obesity does not invariably result in diabetes. Many people who are very obese are able to maintain normal glucose tolerance. Development of diabetes is marked by both insulin resistance and loss of beta cell function.[9] Obesity has been associated with the

[a] Curtis W. and Ann H. Long Department of Family and Community Medicine, University of Missouri, MA306 Medical Sciences Building, DC032.00, Columbia, MO 65212, USA
[b] University of Missouri, Family Medicine Residency Program, MA303 Medical Sciences Building, DC032.00, Columbia, MO 65212, USA
[c] Information Management and Resource Center, M246 Medical Sciences Building, Curtis W. and Ann H. Long Department of Family and Community Medicine, University of Missouri, Columbia, MO 65212, USA
* Corresponding author.
E-mail address: koopmanr@health.missouri.edu (R.J. Koopman).

Prim Care Clin Office Pract 36 (2009) 257–270
doi:10.1016/j.pop.2009.01.006 **primarycare.theclinics.com**
0095-4543/09/$ – see front matter

development of hepatic and renal insulin resistance, even in nondiabetic patients.[10] Genetics also certainly plays a role. Individuals with a family history of diabetes have a reduced beta cell compensatory response to the insulin resistance associated with obesity.[11] Body fat distribution may also play a role. Abdominal fat has a significantly stronger relationship with insulin sensitivity than peripheral fat, accounting for 79% of the variance in insulin sensitivity.[12] Obese diabetics compared with obese nondiabetics have larger abdominal fat cells, which correlate with lower insulin sensitivity and glucose disposal.[13,14] A major function of adipose tissue is to store excess energy as triglycerides under conditions of nutrient excess. In response to prolonged periods of caloric excess, adipose tissue may become overloaded and unable to recruit new fat cells, resulting in adipose tissue hypertrophy and increased ectopic fat deposition. Independent of total body fat, those with larger abdominal fat cells are more insulin resistant and are more likely to develop diabetes.[13,14] It has been hypothesized that free fatty acids released from adipose tissue play a role in hepatic insulin resistance.[10] There is also growing evidence that adipocytes are an endocrine entity and secrete several proteins referred to as adipocytokines in response to a variety of stimuli. These include tumor necrosis factor α, plasminogen-activator inhibitor type 1, adipsin, resistin, leptin, adiponectin, vaspin, and interleukin-6 (IL-6), which have all been linked to insulin resistance.[15–18]

Screening Recommendations

Obesity can be measured in various ways, and there is much debate about which anthropometric index best reflects the risk of diabetes. BMI is usually considered a measure of overall obesity, whereas waist circumference and waist-to-hip ratio both measure central obesity. In prospective studies, BMI, waist circumference, and waist-to-hip ratio were each strongly and independently related to the development of diabetes.[19] Receiver operating characteristic curve analysis indicated that waist circumference and BMI were similar and better than waist-to-hip ratio in predicting type 2 diabetes.[8] National Cholesterol Education Program (NCEP) Adult Treatment Panel III guidelines define abdominal obesity as a waist circumference greater than 102 cm (40 inches) in men and 88 cm (35 inches) in women.[20] There is an additive effect of BMI and waist circumference on predicting the risk of diabetes, with the highest risk observed in men and women with a high BMI in combination with a high waist circumference or waist-to-hip ratio.[19] Both BMI and waist circumference are useful for assessing the risk of diabetes and may be useful to measure when counseling patients on their risk of diabetes and may also prompt screening for diabetes in those with elevated BMI or waist circumference. Currently, the US Preventive Services Task Force (USPSTF) recommends screening for type 2 diabetes in asymptomatic adults with BP greater than 135/80 (grade B) but finds insufficient evidence to recommend screening asymptomatic adults with BP less than 135/80 regardless of the presence of obesity.[21] On the basis of expert opinion, the ADA recommends that health care providers consider screening for type 2 diabetes at 3-year intervals beginning at age 45 years, particularly in those with BMI greater than or equal to 25 kg/m^2. Testing should be considered at a younger age or be performed more frequently in individuals who are overweight and have 1 or more risk factors for diabetes. The ADA recommends screening with fasting plasma glucose (FPG).[4] Recommended diagnostic criteria for diabetes and prediabetes states are presented in **Table 1**.[21]

Prediabetes and Risk of Progression to Diabetes

Impaired glucose states increase the risk of progression to diabetes. IFG is defined by the ADA as FPG greater than or equal to 100 and less than 126 mg/dL, whereas IGT is

Table 1
Diagnostic criteria for normoglycemia, prediabetes, and diabetes

Normoglycemia	IFG or IGT	Diabetes
Fasting glucose <100 mg/dL	FPG ≥100 and <126 (IFG)	FPG ≥126 mg/dL
2-h postload glucose <140 mg/dL	2-h postload glucose ≥140 and <200 mg/dL (IGT)	2-h postload glucose ≥200 mg/dL
—	—	Symptoms of diabetes and casual plasma glucose ≥200 mg/dL

2-h plasma glucose during an oral glucose tolerance test performed as described by the World Health Organization, using a glucose load containing 75 g anhydrous glucose dissolved in water.

Classic symptoms of diabetes include polyuria, polydipsia, and unexplained weight loss.

In the absence of unequivocal hyperglycemia, these criteria should be confirmed by repeat testing on a different day. *Abbreviations:* FPG, fasting plasma glucose; IFG, impaired fasting glucose; IGT, impaired glucose tolerance.

Data from Screening for type 2 diabetes mellitus in adults, topic page. Rockville (MD): U.S. Preventive Services Task Force/Agency for Healthcare Research and Quality; 2008. Available at: http://www.ahrq.gov/clinic/uspstf/uspsdiab.htm. Accessed July 8, 2008.

defined as a 2-hour postload glucose greater than or equal to 140 and less than 200 mg/dL.[4] The crude rates of progression to diabetes during 2 years were 11.5% for patients with IGT compared with 8.4% for those with normal glucose tolerance. Obese subjects with normal glucose tolerance had higher rates of progression to IGT and diabetes than did nonobese subjects.[22]

Interventions to Prevent Progression to Diabetes

Although obesity does increase the risk of developing diabetes, there are interventions that help prevent the progression to diabetes. In the Finnish Diabetes Prevention Study Group, overweight subjects with IGT who were randomized to dietary changes and moderate exercise of at least 30 min/d were able to lose ~4.2 kg by the end of the first year versus 0.8 kg in the control group, reducing their risk of diabetes mellitus (DM) by 58%.[23] In the Diabetes Prevention Program Research Group, lifestyle intervention was found to be superior to metformin and placebo in reducing progression to diabetes among overweight adults with IGT and IFG. Lifestyle intervention involved individualized counseling with the goal of at least 7% weight loss and 150 minutes of physical activity per week. To prevent 1 case of DM during a period of 3 years in those with IGT and IFG, 6.9 persons would have to participate in a lifestyle-intervention program, and 13.9 would have to receive metformin.[24] Intensive lifestyle intervention was also found to produce the greatest improvement in insulin sensitivity and the best preservation of beta cell function after 1 year compared with that of placebo, with metformin results intermediate between those of lifestyle intervention and placebo.[25]

OBESITY AND CARDIOVASCULAR DISEASE

In the past decade, the prevalence of overweight and obesity has increased dramatically. In 1999 to 2000, 65% of US adults were overweight, and 31% of adults were obese and at increased risk for chronic disease.[26] Obesity and its effects on cardiometabolic disease is just 1 area of how obesity can have a profound impact on chronic disease. It has been well understood that obesity is an important risk factor for CVDs, and the role of obesity in predisposing individuals to diabetes, HTN, and other aspects of CVD risk is well established.[27]

One area where obesity and CVD intersect is the metabolic syndrome. The metabolic syndrome—also known as the insulin-resistance syndrome, metabolic syndrome X, and dysmetabolic syndrome—refers to a specific clustering of cardiovascular risk factors in the same individual: abdominal obesity, atherogenic dyslipidemia, elevated blood pressure, insulin resistance, a prothrombotic state, and a proinflammatory state.[28] A formal definition of the syndrome was created by the consensus panel of the NCEP (**Table 2**).[20]

Epidemiology

The prevalence of obesity (BMI $\geq$30 kg/m^2) is increasing in all US population segments, including both genders, children, and adults of all ages, and diverse racial/ethnic groups, across the spectrum of educational attainment. Obesity rates in the United States have risen significantly in recent years: 30% of US adults and 16% of children 6 to 19 years old are obese, and trends suggest that rates will continue to increase.[26,29] Moreover, these statistics are actually a reflection of a global epidemic of obesity.[30]

According to a recent analysis of data from the Third National Health and Nutrition Examination Survey, approximately 47 million Americans (23.7% of the population) have the metabolic syndrome. The prevalence of the metabolic syndrome also increases with age, with a prevalence of greater than 30% in adults older than 40 years, and greater than 40% for adults older than 60 years.[31]

Pathophysiology

There has been continued debate as to whether obesity has a direct impact on CVD or whether its effect is simply mediated by diabetes, HTN, or other intermediate conditions associated with obesity. Recent literature has supported a direct effect of obesity on CVD. Excess abdominal adipose tissue, particularly visceral fat, and excess triglyceride content in liver, skeletal muscle, and heart tissues are associated with hepatic and skeletal muscle insulin resistance, impaired ventricular function, and increased

Table 2
Defining clinical characteristics of the metabolic syndrome

Risk Factors	Defining Clinical Characteristics
Abdominal obesity	Waist circumference
Men	>102 cm (>40 in)
Women	>88 cm (>35 in)
Triglycerides	$\geq$150 mg/dL
HDL cholesterol	
Men	<40 mg/dL
Women	<50 mg/dL
Blood pressure	$\geq$130/$\geq$85 mmHg
Fasting glucose	$\geq$110 mg/dL

Data from National Cholesterol Education Program (NCEP) Expert Panel on Detection, Evaluation, and Treatment of High Blood Cholesterol in Adults (Adult Treatment Panel III). Third Report of the National Cholesterol Education Program (NCEP) Expert Panel on Detection, Evaluation, and Treatment of High Blood Cholesterol in Adults (Adult Treatment Panel III) final report. Circulation 2002;106(25):3143–421.

coronary heart disease (CHD).[32,33] In fact, it has been determined that patients who have the metabolic syndrome and associated obesity have a 3-fold increase in the risk of CHD and stroke.[34]

Obesity and Its Direct Cardiac Effect

Obesity, in and of itself, is associated with abnormalities in cardiac structure and function. Obesity is associated with an increase in total blood volume and cardiac output and a decrease in peripheral vascular resistance.[32] Essentially, an obese person at any given level of activity will have a greater workload than that of a nonobese individual. In this setting, ventricular filling pressures are elevated, which causes increased wall stress, dysfunction, and hypertrophy.[35] This subsequently can lead to left-ventricular hypertrophy and left-atrial enlargement, with the potential to develop arrhythmias, cardiomyopathy, and cardiac events.

Obesity and Its Effect on Noncardiac Organs and Subsequent Cardiovascular Disease

CHD in obese persons may also result from indirect strain on the heart. It has been suggested that the limited ability of subcutaneous fat depots to store excess energy results in "overflow" of chemical energy to intra-abdominal adipose tissues and ectopic sites, such as the liver and skeletal muscle.[36] Excessive ectopic fat accumulation then can cause metabolic dysfunction in organs, which will go on to cause insulin resistance and other comorbidities of CVD.[36]

Obesity and Inflammation

Obesity is associated with an increase in circulating inflammatory markers, including C-reactive protein (CRP) and cytokines, such as IL-6, IL-18, and P-selectin.[37] Adipose tissue itself is a likely source of these excess cytokines, and IL-6 stimulates the production of CRP by the liver.[38] The increase in inflammatory markers is associated with insulin resistance and is likely an important predictor of atherosclerotic events.[39] Obesity has also been associated with oxidative stress in members of the Framingham cohort.[40] Other risk factors associated with obesity, for example, hyperglycemia, insulin resistance, dyslipidemia, diet, and HTN, could also increase inflammation.[41] The vascular endothelium, as well, plays an important role in cardiovascular homeostasis by modulating vascular tone, inhibiting monocyte and platelet adhesion, and maintaining fibrinolytic balance. In obesity, the endothelium is exposed to mechanical forces and other cardiovascular risk factors that can alter vascular structure and function, thus resulting in disease and subsequent cardiovascular events.[42]

Associations of and Contributions to Cardiovascular Disease

Moving from the molecular basis of disease to more patient-oriented outcomes, recent studies have demonstrated the relationship between obesity and CVD. The overall hazard ratios for all-cause and CVD mortality in persons with the metabolic syndrome as compared with those in persons without it were 1.44 and 2.26 in men and 1.38 and 2.78 in women after adjustment for age, blood cholesterol levels, and smoking.[43] In a prospective, population-based study among middle-aged Finnish men, waist-to-hip ratio, waist circumference, and BMI as continuous variables were directly associated with the risk of CHD. On average, each 1 standard deviation increase in any of the measures discussed here increased the cardiovascular risk more than 20%.[44] Similarly, among men presenting with acute myocardial infarction, long-term, all-cause mortality was associated with increased abdominal obesity, even after controlling for conditions associated with visceral adiposity, including HTN and diabetes.[45] These results suggest a possible direct effect of obesity on all-cause mortality.

Ample evidence supports the indirect effects of obesity on CVD as well. HTN itself is about more than 2 times more prevalent in obese subjects than in lean adult men and women.[46] Weight gain in young people is a potent risk factor for subsequent development of HTN.[47] Obesity in adolescents and young adults accelerates the progression of atherosclerosis decades before the appearance of clinical manifestations.[48] According to a meta-analysis by Bogers and colleagues,[49] adverse effects of overweight on blood pressure and cholesterol levels could account for about 45% of the increased risk of CHD.

Management and Benefits

Management of the metabolic syndrome consists primarily of 2 strategies: modification or reversal of the root causes, including weight reduction and increased physical activity, and direct treatment of the metabolic risk factors, including atherogenic dyslipidemia, elevated blood pressure, the prothrombotic state, and underlying insulin resistance.[28] Many would argue that the metabolic syndrome is a useful conceptual and clinical grouping, but that, for the purposes of prognosis and therapy, it is no more significant than the sum of its parts.[50]

Weight reduction and increased physical activity are areas that are more easily discussed than achieved. The CDC recommends behavior changes, including an increase in physical activity and intake of vegetables and fruits.[51] The USPSTF found insufficient evidence to recommend brief counseling for overweight adults, but they did recommend high-intensity counseling for dietary change and exercise to obese adults.[52] Lifestyle interventions with a weight-reducing diet and regular exercise greatly decrease metabolic CHD risk factors within adult obese populations.[53]

Bariatric surgery may be another weight loss strategy for the very obese. Data from the Swedish Obese Subjects study showed that an average weight loss of 33% at 2 years after bariatric surgical intervention decreased serum triglyceride concentrations and increased serum HDL-C (cholesterol) concentrations.[54]

Prevention of obesity is a key strategy in producing improved health for populations. Prevention requires both structural approaches (community-level changes and policies at local, state, and national levels) and individually oriented approaches. These approaches must be carefully formulated in consideration of the ethnic, cultural, and social embedment of many of the factors that determine obesity.[28]

OBESITY AND POLYCYSTIC OVARY SYNDROME

PCOS is a heterogeneous syndrome occurring in women characterized by anovulation, which often presents as menstrual irregularity and/or infertility, and hyperandrogenism, presenting as hirsutism, acne, and male-pattern balding. Important metabolic associations include central obesity, insulin resistance, and dyslipidemia. Obesity and PCOS seem to often have synergistic deleterious effects on metabolic parameters for women with this syndrome. Treatment should be individualized to reflect patient concerns, desired fertility, and metabolic consequences.

Definition of the Polycystic Ovary Syndrome

Although a directed history and physical examination will likely suggest the possibility of PCOS, diagnosis of PCOS can be somewhat challenging for several reasons. First, PCOS is a syndrome, a phenotype. As such, there is no 1 definitive diagnostic test. Second, since PCOS is a familial disease, patients may under-report symptoms.

If a patient's mother had a similar pattern of hirsutism and also had trouble with infrequent heavy periods, then the patient's symptoms may be felt to be something that "runs in the family" rather than a potential disease entity whose symptoms they should report to their doctor. Third, disease manifestations may vary throughout life. Finally, there are more than 1 set of diagnostic criteria, as represented in **Table 3**.[55–57]

Notably, only the Rotterdam criteria include polycystic ovaries in the criteria, although they are not necessary for diagnosis if the other 2 criteria are present. The presence of polycystic ovarian morphology alone does not reliably predict the development of PCOS; in fact, half of ovaries with polycystic morphology resolve with time.[58]

Differential Diagnosis and Diagnostic Workup

The differential diagnosis of PCOS includes other hormonal disorders with similar clinical features, especially those with manifestations of hyperandrogenism and anovulation, including nonclassical congenital adrenal hyperplasia, Cushing's syndrome, androgen-secreting tumors, thyroid disorders, premature ovarian failure, hyperprolactinemia, and acromegaly.[56] The likelihood of many of these conditions can be evaluated clinically. Although clinicians may want to examine the possibility of nonclassical congenital adrenal hyperplasia by checking a 17-hydroxyprogesterone level, routine laboratory testing for a panel of conditions may not be warranted. For example, mild elevations in prolactin level may be seen in many women with PCOS.[56] In addition to the clinical assessment of hyperandrogenism, a practical approach to laboratory assessment of hyperandrogenism is to measure dehydroepiandrosterone sulfate and free testosterone.[59] Mild elevations of these hormones can be expected in the woman with PCOS, whereas high levels may suggest an androgen-producing tumor of the ovary or adrenal gland.[59]

Epidemiology of PCOS

The prevalence of PCOS in an unselected population of the Southeastern United States was 6.6%, with similar prevalence rates among white and black women.[60] A similar prevalence, 6.5%, was found among unselected white women in Spain.[61] However, among select populations, PCOS prevalence is much higher; clinicians can expect to find rates of 28.3% in otherwise unselected overweight and obese

Table 3
Diagnostic criteria for Polycystic Ovary Syndrome

NIH Criteria (1990)	Rotterdam Criteria (2003)	AACE Criteria (2005)
Ovulatory dysfunction	Oligomenorrhea or amenorrhea[a]	Irregular menses and anovulation with onset at puberty
Hyperandrogenism clinically or by laboratory testing	Hyperandrogenism clinically or by laboratory testing[a]	Hyperandrogenism by laboratory testing
—	Polycystic ovaries on ultrasonography[a]	—
Exclusion of other hormonal disorders with similar clinical features	Exclusion of other hormonal disorders with similar clinical features	Exclusion of other hormonal disorders with similar clinical features

Abbreviations: AACE, The American Association of Clinical Endocrinologists; NIH, National Institutes of Health.
[a] 2 of these 3 criteria for diagnosis.

premenopausal white women, 26.7% in premenopausal women with type 2 diabetes, and 35% and 40% among premenopausal sisters and mothers of women with PCOS, respectively.[62–64]

Pathophysiology and the Role of Obesity

Obesity, a common and important part of the PCOS phenotype, has increased in the United States during the last 2 decades.[26,65] However, although the degree of obesity among women with PCOS has increased during the last 2 decades, there has been only a modest and nonsignificant increase in the prevalence of PCOS among an unselected population of women during that same time.[66] These findings suggest that the risk of developing PCOS is only modestly increased with obesity, whereas women with PCOS are subject to the same environmental influences that promote obesity in our society.[66]

Insulin resistance is more common among women with PCOS than that among age- and BMI-matched women without PCOS.[67] Although increasing BMI is associated with increasing insulin resistance in women without PCOS, those with PCOS develop an even greater degree of insulin resistance as BMI increases.[67–69] Both lean and obese women with PCOS showed a predilection for truncal obesity in their body fat distribution, with obese women with PCOS having a very similar fat distribution to women with type 2 diabetes.[70]

Hyperandrogenism among women with PCOS does not correlate with the degree of insulin resistance, suggesting that this may represent independent pathophysiologic factors.[68] PCOS and obesity have a synergistic deleterious effect on glucose tolerance; it is likely that PCOS is associated with a unique disorder of insulin action.[67]

Perhaps concomitant with the role of insulin resistance, women with PCOS have been found to have a variety of other metabolic abnormalities prompting some to suggest the moniker Syndrome XX for PCOS.[71] The metabolic syndrome is more prevalent in women with PCOS, with prevalence rates of 43% to 46% among newly diagnosed women with PCOS.[72,73] Women with PCOS are approximately twice as likely (46.4 vs 22.8%) to have the metabolic syndrome as do age-matched controls and are also more likely to have abdominal obesity, low HDL-C, and high blood pressure.[73] After adjusting for BMI, adolescent girls with PCOS are 4.5 times more likely to have the metabolic syndrome than do age-matched girls without PCOS.[74] Other metabolic abnormalities have been found in excess among women with PCOS, including IGT, type 2 diabetes, elevated total cholesterol, elevated triglycerides, early atherosclerosis as measured by carotid intima-media thickness, and endothelial dysfunction as measured by flow-mediated dilation.[75–77] Additionally, PCOS has been associated with genomic variants related to increased oxidative stress, insulin resistance, and hyperandrogenism.[78]

Metabolic Outcomes

By the fourth decade of life, 35% of women with PCOS have IGT, and 10% have type 2 diabetes.[76] Women with PCOS are at a significantly increased risk for IGT at all weights and at a young age.[79] PCOS is also associated with an increased prevalence of obstructive sleep apnea, again in excess of the prevalence among age- and weight-matched controls.[80] Although data on the association of PCOS with subsequent cardiovascular events are lacking, women with PCOS have been shown to have increased prevalence of HTN, abnormal lipid profiles, signs of early atherosclerosis, increased left atrial size, increased left ventricular mass index, and lower left ventricular ejection fracture, in addition to a greater prevalence of the metabolic syndrome.[72,73,75,77,81,82] Taken together with the evidence for increased risk of IGT and diabetes, it is likely that women with PCOS have excess CVD and events over and above otherwise similar obese women without PCOS.

Fertility and Pregnancy Outcomes

PCOS is the most common cause of anovulatory infertility.[83,84] Women with PCOS who do become pregnant have an increased risk of spontaneous abortion.[85] As might be anticipated, gestational DM has an increased prevalence in women with PCOS, as high as 20%.[86] Similar to other metabolic parameters, gestational diabetes is increased most in obese women with PCOS, again suggesting a synergistic relationship between PCOS and obesity.[86] Women with PCOS also have a higher risk for other pregnancy complications, including pregnancy-induced HTN, pre-eclampsia, and preterm birth.[87]

Treatment

The treatment of PCOS is multifaceted, reflecting the heterogeneity of the disorder and the several desired outcomes of treatment. Treatment of hirsutism involves the use of local depilatory treatments. The metabolic profile of PCOS can be improved with lifestyle modification, weight loss, and metformin.[73] Anovulatory cycles, the hallmark of PCOS, which lead to both menstrual irregularity and infertility, are also improved by weight loss and metformin.[88–91] In the treatment of infertility, metformin plus the ovulation-inducing agent clomiphene is more effective than clomiphene alone.[89–91] Weight loss through lifestyle modification is, therefore, a recommended main or adjunct treatment for almost all PCOS treatment objectives.

REFERENCES

1. Cowie CC, Rust KF, Byrd-Holt DD, et al. Prevalence of diabetes and impaired fasting glucose in adults in the U.S. population: National Health And Nutrition Examination Survey 1999–2002. Diabetes Care 2006;29(6):1263–8.
2. Mainous AG III, Baker R, Koopman RJ, et al. Impact of the population at risk of diabetes on projections of diabetes burden in the United States: an epidemic on the way. Diabetologia 2007;50(5):934–40.
3. Hu FB, Manson JE, Stampfer MJ, et al. Diet, lifestyle, and the risk of type 2 diabetes mellitus in women. N Engl J Med 2001;345(11):790–7.
4. American Diabetes Association. Standards of medical care in diabetes–2008. Diabetes Care 2008;31(Suppl 1):S12–54.
5. Centers for Disease Control and Prevention (CDC). Prevalence of overweight and obesity among adults with diagnosed diabetes–United States, 1988–1994 and 1999-2002. MMWR Morb Mortal Wkly Rep 2004;53(45):1066–8.
6. Weinstein AR, Sesso HD, Lee IM, et al. Relationship of physical activity vs body mass index with type 2 diabetes in women. JAMA 2004;292(10):1188–94.
7. Patterson RE, Frank LL, Kristal AR, et al. A comprehensive examination of health conditions associated with obesity in older adults. Am J Prev Med 2004;27(5): 385–90.
8. Wang Y, Rimm EB, Stampfer MJ, et al. Comparison of abdominal adiposity and overall obesity in predicting risk of type 2 diabetes among men. Am J Clin Nutr 2005;81(3):555–63.
9. Burns N, Finucane FM, Hatunic M, et al. Early-onset type 2 diabetes in obese white subjects is characterised by a marked defect in beta cell insulin secretion, severe insulin resistance and a lack of response to aerobic exercise training. Diabetologia 2007;50(7):1500–8.

10. Paquot N, Scheen AJ, Dirlewanger M, et al. Hepatic insulin resistance in obese non-diabetic subjects and in type 2 diabetic patients. Obes Res 2002;10(3): 129–34.
11. Elbein SC, Wegner K, Kahn SE. Reduced beta-cell compensation to the insulin resistance associated with obesity in members of Caucasian familial type 2 diabetic kindreds. Diabetes Care 2000;23(2):221–7.
12. Carey DG, Jenkins AB, Campbell LV, et al. Abdominal fat and insulin resistance in normal and overweight women: direct measurements reveal a strong relationship in subjects at both low and high risk of NIDDM. Diabetes 1996;45(5):633–8.
13. Dubois SG, Heilbronn LK, Smith SR, et al. Decreased expression of adipogenic genes in obese subjects with type 2 diabetes. Obesity (Silver spring) 2006;14(9): 1543–52.
14. Weyer C, Foley JE, Bogardus C, et al. Enlarged subcutaneous abdominal adipocyte size, but not obesity itself, predicts type II diabetes independent of insulin resistance. Diabetologia 2000;43(12):1498–506.
15. Jazet IM, Pijl H, Meinders AE. Adipose tissue as an endocrine organ: impact on insulin resistance. Neth J Med 2003;61(6):194–212.
16. Kim C, Park J, Park J, et al. Comparison of body fat composition and serum adiponectin levels in diabetic obesity and non-diabetic obesity. Obesity 2006; 14(7):1164–71.
17. Weyer C, Funahashi T, Tanaka S, et al. Hypoadiponectinemia in obesity and type 2 diabetes: close association with insulin resistance and hyperinsulinemia. J Clin Endocrinol Metab 2001;86(5):1930–5.
18. Youn BS, Kloting N, Kratzsch J, et al. Serum vaspin concentrations in human obesity and type 2 diabetes. Diabetes 2008;57(2):372–7.
19. Meisinger C, Doring A, Thorand B, et al. Body fat distribution and risk of type 2 diabetes in the general population: are there differences between men and women? The MONICA/KORA Augsburg cohort study. Am J Clin Nutr 2006; 84(3):483–9.
20. National Cholesterol Education Program (NCEP) Expert Panel on Detection, Evaluation, and Treatment of High Blood Cholesterol in Adults (Adult Treatment Panel III). Third Report of the National Cholesterol Education Program (NCEP) Expert Panel on Detection, Evaluation, and Treatment of High Blood Cholesterol in Adults (Adult Treatment Panel III) final report. Circulation 2002;106(25):3143–421.
21. Screening for type 2 diabetes mellitus in adults, topic page. Rockville (MD): U.S. Preventive Services Task Force/Agency for Healthcare Research and Quality; 2008. Available at: http://www.ahrq.gov/clinic/uspstf/uspsdiab.htm. Accessed July 8, 2008.
22. Ko GT, Chan JC, Chow CC, et al. Effects of obesity on the conversion from normal glucose tolerance to diabetes in Hong Kong Chinese. Obes Res 2004;12(6):889–95.
23. Tuomilehto J, Lindstrom J, Eriksson JG, et al. Prevention of type 2 diabetes mellitus by changes in lifestyle among subjects with impaired glucose tolerance. N Engl J Med 2001;344(18):1343–50.
24. Knowler WC, Barrett-Connor E, Fowler SE, et al. Reduction in the incidence of type 2 diabetes with lifestyle intervention or metformin. N Engl J Med 2002; 346(6):393–403.
25. Kitabchi AE, Temprosa M, Knowler WC, et al. Role of insulin secretion and sensitivity in the evolution of type 2 diabetes in the diabetes prevention program: effects of lifestyle intervention and metformin. Diabetes 2005;54(8):2404–14.
26. Flegal KM, Carroll MD, Ogden CL, et al. Prevalence and trends in obesity among US adults, 1999–2000. JAMA 2002;288(14):1723–7.

27. Klein S, Allison DB, Heymsfield SB, et al. Waist circumference and cardiometabolic risk: a consensus statement from shaping America's health: Association for Weight Management and Obesity Prevention; NAASO, the Obesity Society; the American Society for Nutrition; and the American Diabetes Association. Diabetes Care 2007;30(6):1647–52.
28. Smith SC Jr, Clark LT, Cooper RS, et al. Discovering the full spectrum of cardiovascular disease: Minority Health Summit 2003: report of the Obesity, Metabolic Syndrome, and Hypertension Writing Group. Circulation 2005;111(10):e134–9.
29. Ogden CL, Flegal KM, Carroll MD, et al. Prevalence and trends in overweight among US children and adolescents, 1999–2000. JAMA 2002;288(14):1728–32.
30. Obesity: preventing and managing the global epidemic. Report of a WHO consultation. World Health Organ Tech Rep Ser 2000;894:1–253.
31. Ford ES, Giles WH, Dietz WH. Prevalence of the metabolic syndrome among US adults: findings from the third National Health and Nutrition Examination Survey. JAMA 2002;287(3):356–9.
32. Alpert MA. Obesity cardiomyopathy: pathophysiology and evolution of the clinical syndrome. Am J Med Sci 2001;321(4):225–36.
33. Pouliot MC, Despres JP, Lemieux S, et al. Waist circumference and abdominal sagittal diameter: best simple anthropometric indexes of abdominal visceral adipose tissue accumulation and related cardiovascular risk in men and women. Am J Cardiol 1994;73(7):460–8.
34. Isomaa B, Almgren P, Tuomi T, et al. Cardiovascular morbidity and mortality associated with the metabolic syndrome. Diabetes Care 2001;24(4):683–9.
35. Ku CS, Lin SL, Wang DJ, et al. Left ventricular filling in young normotensive obese adults. Am J Cardiol 1994;73(8):613–5.
36. Seppala-Lindroos A, Vehkavaara S, Hakkinen AM, et al. Fat accumulation in the liver is associated with defects in insulin suppression of glucose production and serum free fatty acids independent of obesity in normal men. J Clin Endocrinol Metab 2002;87(7):3023–8.
37. Ziccardi P, Nappo F, Giugliano G, et al. Reduction of inflammatory cytokine concentrations and improvement of endothelial functions in obese women after weight loss over one year. Circulation 2002;105(7):804–9.
38. Mohamed-Ali V, Goodrick S, Rawesh A, et al. Subcutaneous adipose tissue releases interleukin-6, but not tumor necrosis factor-alpha, in vivo. J Clin Endocrinol Metab 1997;82(12):4196–200.
39. Ridker PM. High-sensitivity C-reactive protein: potential adjunct for global risk assessment in the primary prevention of cardiovascular disease. Circulation 2001;103(13):1813–8.
40. Keaney JF Jr, Larson MG, Vasan RS, et al. Obesity and systemic oxidative stress: clinical correlates of oxidative stress in the Framingham Study. Arterioscler Thromb Vasc Biol 2003;23(3):434–9.
41. Engstrom G, Hedblad B, Stavenow L, et al. Incidence of obesity-associated cardiovascular disease is related to inflammation-sensitive plasma proteins: a population-based cohort study. Arterioscler Thromb Vasc Biol 2004;24(8):1498–502.
42. Davy KP, Hall JE. Obesity and hypertension: two epidemics or one? Am J Physiol Regul Integr Comp Physiol 2004;286(5):R803–13.
43. Hu G, Qiao Q, Tuomilehto J, et al. Prevalence of the metabolic syndrome and its relation to all-cause and cardiovascular mortality in nondiabetic European men and women. Arch Intern Med 2004;164(10):1066–76.

44. Lakka HM, Lakka TA, Tuomilehto J, et al. Abdominal obesity is associated with increased risk of acute coronary events in men. Eur Heart J 2002;23(9):706–13.
45. Kragelund C, Hassager C, Hildebrandt P, et al. Impact of obesity on long-term prognosis following acute myocardial infarction. Int J Cardiol 2005;98(1):123–31.
46. Brown CD, Higgins M, Donato KA, et al. Body mass index and the prevalence of hypertension and dyslipidemia. Obes Res 2000;8(9):605–19.
47. Clinical Guidelines on the Identification, Evaluation, and Treatment of Overweight and Obesity in Adults–The Evidence Report. National Institutes of Health. Obes Res 1998;6(Suppl 2):51S–209S.
48. McGill HC Jr, McMahan CA, Malcom GT, et al. Relation of glycohemoglobin and adiposity to atherosclerosis in youth. Pathobiological Determinants of Atherosclerosis in Youth (PDAY) Research Group. Arterioscler Thromb Vasc Biol 1995;15(4):431–40.
49. Bogers RP, Bemelmans WJ, Hoogenveen RT, et al. Association of overweight with increased risk of coronary heart disease partly independent of blood pressure and cholesterol levels: a meta-analysis of 21 cohort studies including more than 300 000 persons. Arch Intern Med 2007;167(16):1720–8.
50. Kahn R. Metabolic syndrome (emperor) wears no clothes. Diabetes Care 2006; 29(7):1693–5.
51. Centers for Disease Control and Prevention (U.S.). Physical Activity and Good Nutrition: Essential Elements to Prevent Chronic Diseases and Obesity At A Glance 2008. Centers for Disease Control and Prevention (U.S.); 2008. Available at: http://cdc.gov/nccdphp/publications/aag/dnpa.htm. Accessed July 30, 2008.
52. McTigue KM, Harris R, Hemphill B, et al. Screening and interventions for obesity in adults: summary of the evidence for the U.S. Preventive Services Task Force. Ann Intern Med 2003;139(11):933–49.
53. Villareal DT, Miller BV III, Banks M, et al. Effect of lifestyle intervention on metabolic coronary heart disease risk factors in obese older adults. Am J Clin Nutr 2006;84(6):1317–23.
54. Sjostrom CD, Lissner L, Wedel H, et al. Reduction in incidence of diabetes, hypertension and lipid disturbances after intentional weight loss induced by bariatric surgery: the SOS Intervention Study. Obes Res 1999;7(5):477–84.
55. American College of Obstetricians and Gynecologists. ACOG practice bulletin. Polycystic ovary syndrome. Number 41, December 2002. Int J Gynaecol Obstet 2003;80(3):335–48.
56. Rotterdam ESHRE-ASRM-Sponsored PCOS Consensus Workshop Group. Revised 2003 consensus on diagnostic criteria and long-term health risks related to polycystic ovary syndrome. Fertil Steril 2004;81(1):19–25.
57. Polycystic Ovary Syndrome Writing Committee. American Association of Clinical Endocrinologists Position Statement on Metabolic and Cardiovascular Consequences of Polycystic Ovary Syndrome. Endocr Pract 2005;11(2):126–34.
58. Murphy MK, Hall JE, Adams JM, et al. Polycystic ovarian morphology in normal women does not predict the development of polycystic ovary syndrome. J Clin Endocrinol Metab 2006;91(10):3878–84.
59. Chang RJ. A practical approach to the diagnosis of polycystic ovary syndrome. Am J Obstet Gynecol 2004;191(3):713–7.
60. Azziz R, Woods KS, Reyna R, et al. The prevalence and features of the polycystic ovary syndrome in an unselected population. J Clin Endocrinol Metab 2004; 89(6):2745–9.
61. Asuncion M, Calvo RM, San Millan JL, et al. A prospective study of the prevalence of the polycystic ovary syndrome in unselected Caucasian women from Spain. J Clin Endocrinol Metab 2000;85(7):2434–8.

62. Alvarez-Blasco F, Botella-Carretero JI, San Millan JL, et al. Prevalence and characteristics of the polycystic ovary syndrome in overweight and obese women. Arch Intern Med 2006;166(19):2081–6.
63. Kahsar-Miller MD, Nixon C, Boots LR, et al. Prevalence of polycystic ovary syndrome (PCOS) in first-degree relatives of patients with PCOS. Fertil Steril 2001;75(1):53–8.
64. Peppard HR, Marfori J, Iuorno MJ, et al. Prevalence of polycystic ovary syndrome among premenopausal women with type 2 diabetes. Diabetes Care 2001;24(6): 1050–2.
65. Mokdad AH, Serdula MK, Dietz WH, et al. The spread of the obesity epidemic in the United States, 1991-1998. JAMA 1999;282(16):1519–22.
66. Yildiz BO, Knochenhauer ES, Azziz R. Impact of obesity on the risk for polycystic ovary syndrome. J Clin Endocrinol Metab 2008;93(1):162–8.
67. Dunaif A, Segal KR, Futterweit W, et al. Profound peripheral insulin resistance, independent of obesity, in polycystic ovary syndrome. Diabetes 1989;38(9):1165–74.
68. Rittmaster RS, Deshwal N, Lehman L. The role of adrenal hyperandrogenism, insulin resistance, and obesity in the pathogenesis of polycystic ovarian syndrome. J Clin Endocrinol Metab 1993;76(5):1295–300.
69. Acien P, Quereda F, Matallin P, et al. Insulin, androgens, and obesity in women with and without polycystic ovary syndrome: a heterogeneous group of disorders. Fertility & Sterility 1999;72(1):32–40.
70. Horejsi R, Moller R, Rackl S, et al. Android subcutaneous adipose tissue topography in lean and obese women suffering from PCOS: comparison with type 2 diabetic women. Am J Phys Anthropol 2004;124(3):275–81.
71. Sam S, Dunaif A. Polycystic ovary syndrome: syndrome XX? Trends Endocrinol Metab 2003;14(8):365–70.
72. Apridonidze T, Essah PA, Iuorno MJ, et al. Prevalence and characteristics of the metabolic syndrome in women with polycystic ovary syndrome. J Clin Endocrinol Metab 2005;90(4):1929–35.
73. Glueck CJ, Papanna R, Wang P, et al. Incidence and treatment of metabolic syndrome in newly referred women with confirmed polycystic ovarian syndrome. Metabolism 2003;52(7):908–15.
74. Coviello AD, Legro RS, Dunaif A. Adolescent girls with polycystic ovary syndrome have an increased risk of the metabolic syndrome associated with increasing androgen levels independent of obesity and insulin resistance. J Clin Endocrinol Metab 2006;91(2):492–7.
75. Carmina E, Orio F, Palomba S, et al. Endothelial dysfunction in PCOS: role of obesity and adipose hormones. Am J Med 2006;119(4):356.
76. Ehrmann DA, Barnes RB, Rosenfield RL, et al. Prevalence of impaired glucose tolerance and diabetes in women with polycystic ovary syndrome. Diabetes Care 1999;22(1):141–6.
77. Meyer C, McGrath BP, Teede HJ. Overweight women with polycystic ovary syndrome have evidence of subclinical cardiovascular disease. J Clin Endocrinol Metab 2005;90(10):5711–6.
78. San Millan JL, Corton M, Villuendas G, et al. Association of the polycystic ovary syndrome with genomic variants related to insulin resistance, type 2 diabetes mellitus, and obesity. J Clin Endocrinol Metab 2004;89(6):2640–6.
79. Legro RS, Kunselman AR, Dodson WC, et al. Prevalence and predictors of risk for type 2 diabetes mellitus and impaired glucose tolerance in polycystic ovary syndrome: a prospective, controlled study in 254 affected women. J Clin Endocrinol Metab 1999;84(1):165–9.

80. Fogel RB, Malhotra A, Pillar G, et al. Increased prevalence of obstructive sleep apnea syndrome in obese women with polycystic ovary syndrome. J Clin Endocrinol Metab 2001;86(3):1175–80.
81. Orio F Jr, Palomba S, Spinelli L, et al. The cardiovascular risk of young women with polycystic ovary syndrome: an observational, analytical, prospective case-control study. J Clin Endocrinol Metab 2004;89(8):3696–701.
82. Mahabeer S, Naidoo C, Norman RJ, et al. Metabolic profiles and lipoprotein lipid concentrations in non-obese and obese patients with polycystic ovarian disease. Horm Metab Res 1990;22(10):537–40.
83. Homburg R. Polycystic ovary syndrome - from gynaecological curiosity to multisystem endocrinopathy. Humanit Rep 1996;11(1):29–39.
84. Costello MF, Eden JA. A systematic review of the reproductive system effects of metformin in patients with polycystic ovary syndrome. Fertility & Sterility 2003; 79(1):1–13.
85. Homburg R. Pregnancy complications in PCOS. Best Pract Res Clin Endocrinol Metab 2006;20(2):281–92.
86. Mikola M, Hiilesmaa V, Halttunen M, et al. Obstetric outcome in women with polycystic ovarian syndrome. Hum Reprod 2001;16(2):226–9.
87. Boomsma CM, Eijkemans MJ, Hughes EG, et al. A meta-analysis of pregnancy outcomes in women with polycystic ovary syndrome. Hum Reprod Update 2006;12(6):673–83.
88. Al Azemi M, Omu FE, Omu AE. The effect of obesity on the outcome of infertility management in women with polycystic ovary syndrome. Arch Gynecol Obstet 2004;270(4):205–10.
89. Barbieri RL. Metformin for the treatment of polycystic ovary syndrome. Obstet Gynecol 2003;101(4):785–93.
90. Creanga AA, Bradley HM, McCormick C, et al. Use of metformin in polycystic ovary syndrome: a meta-analysis. Obstet Gynecol 2008;111(4):959–68.
91. Lord JM, Flight IH, Norman RJ. Metformin in polycystic ovary syndrome: systematic review and meta-analysis. BMJ 2003;327(7421):951–3.

Comorbidities of Obesity

Kavitha Bhat Schelbert, MD, MS

KEYWORDS

- Obesity • Comorbidities • Adiposity • Malignancy
- Insulin resistance

When chronic excessive caloric intake occurs, the body develops metabolic, cellular, and mechanical adaptations. These adaptations sometimes manifest into particular clinical diseases and conditions, causing significant morbidity and mortality. In this review, we briefly discuss the major adaptations that can develop when increased intake and decreased expenditure occur. Next, we evaluate the changes in metabolism, such as insulin resistance, proinflammatory mediation, dyslipidemia, and fatty acid release. Finally, we discuss how these changes manifest into disease, dysfunction, and sometimes mortality in certain obese patients.

PATHOPHYSIOLOGY OF ADIPOSITY

Energy Homeostasis

The obesity epidemic is driven by an imbalance between energy intake, which is primarily behaviorally dependent, and energy expenditure, which is, in part, involuntary. This excess energy intake must be stored as fat in adipocytes, which are part of the body's largest endocrine unit. When energy expenditure is required, fat within the adipocytes is oxidized to release free fatty acids (FFAs) for gluconeogenesis and energy use.[1–3]

Pathophysiology of Increased Inactivity and Increased Energy Expenditure

Relatively little is known about the physiology of inactivity. Yet nonexercise activity thermogenesis comprises a greater component of total energy expenditure than that of exercise. Hamilton and colleagues[3] propose a conceptual framework that considers sitting and other sedentary behaviors quite distinct from activity and may differentially affect cellular responses that are implicated in the development of metabolic risk factors for diabetes and heart disease. They propose that any type of brief, yet frequent, muscular contraction throughout the day may be necessary to "short circuit" unhealthy molecular signals causing metabolic diseases. Studies examining

Department of Family Medicine, University of Pittsburgh School of Medicine, 3518 Fifth Avenue, Pittsburgh, PA 15261, USA
E-mail address: schelbertkb@upmc.edu

Prim Care Clin Office Pract 36 (2009) 271–285
doi:10.1016/j.pop.2009.01.009 **primarycare.theclinics.com**
0095-4543/09/$ – see front matter

the cellular regulation of skeletal muscle lipoprotein lipase (LPL), a protein important for controlling plasma triglyceride catabolism, high-density lipoprotein (HDL) cholesterol, and other metabolic risk factors revealed a potential molecular basis to maintain high levels of daily low-intensity and intermittent activity. Reductions in spontaneous standing and ambulatory time affected LPL regulation much more than adding vigorous exercise training to normal levels of nonexercise activity. Inactivity initiated unique cellular responses, causing metabolic dysregulation.[3]

Exercise and activity behaviors may conversely promote separate cellular signals that promote good health. Importantly, the most potent physical activity mechanism that determines risk factor development is the maintenance of a high volume of daily, intermittent, low-intensity, postural and ambulatory activity.[2,3]

Development of the Pathologic Adipocyte

Adipose tissue is the largest endocrine organ in the body. The development of potentially pathologic adipocytes, the cellular unit of adipose tissue, may confer risk upon those who gain weight. Yet pathogenic adipocyte formation is not the only mechanism in play. The variability with which fat weight gain causes metabolic disease depends on several factors, including *how* fat is stored (in new adipocytes—by adipogenesis, vs by pathogenic hypertrophy of existing adipocytes); *where* fat is stored (visceral, subcutaneous, or ectopic depots), and also *how adipocytes signal* and interact with other organs.[2,4] The development of enlarged adipocytes is hypothesized to be related to the relative inability of these groups, including Asians and Native Americans, to develop new fat cells or adipogenesis independent of BMI.[2] Ideally when a positive caloric balance occurs, new adipocytes are generated from preadipocytes to store FFAs. The key determinant of comorbid disease in obesity may not be the amount of fat that is stored during positive caloric balance but the manner in which it is stored. When adipocyte hypertrophy occurs, metabolic disturbances seem to develop, whereas during adipogenesis adipocyte hyperplasia may result in a metabolically stable state.

Without the available adipose tissue precursors, FFA oxidation is limited, and lipotoxicity from circulating FFAs develops. What is more, FFAs can form depots in other sites, such as the liver and muscle, causing local and systemic insulin resistance.[1,4,5] If physiology to maintain normal adiposity is depleted from under- or malnutrition, then lipodystrophy causes hormonal, reproductive, and developmental abnormalities. Excess adiposity conversely provides inflammatory secretagogues, particularly from central visceral fat depots, which enhance insulin resistance and the circulation of FFAs.[6]

THE PATHOLOGIC ADIPOCYTE CAUSES METABOLIC DYSREGULATION

Simply put, obesity causes disease and dysfunction through 2 specific mechanisms: the interaction of hormones and regulatory cytokines produced by fat cells or adipocytes, and the mechanical adjustments associated with increased body mass. The clinical manifestations thus listed will occur in relation to the pathophysiologic mechanisms that cause that condition.

Abdominal Obesity and Adipokines: A Starting Point

Substantial evidence suggests that the relationship of obesity to metabolic dysfunction lies not in BMI but rather in abdominal obesity.[7,8] Based on studies using magnetic resonance imaging, metabolic dysfunction is correlated with intra-abdominal or visceral adipose tissue and ectopic fat deposition, not subcutaneous abdominal fat.[7] Adipocytes within the visceral adipose tissue cause the release of several adipokines, including adiponectin, interleukin-6 (IL-6), tumor necrosis factor-alpha (TNF-α), C-reactive protein (CRP), leptin, and resistin. These adipokines are associated with specific metabolic dysfunctions, including insulin resistance, proinflammatory mediation, and excessive fatty acid production (**Fig. 1**).[1,6,9]

Adiponectin

One of the most important regulators of metabolic dysregulation is adiponectin. Adiponectin is the most abundant product of adipocytes. Adiponectin levels in systemic circulation act to improve insulin sensitivity and reduce inflammation. It modulates glucose and FFA metabolism. Low levels of adiponectin, a state that occurs in the presence of the dysfunctional adipocyte, promote the development of insulin resistance, type 2 diabetes mellitus, and atherosclerosis. Conversely, with chronic caloric restriction, adiponectin levels rise.[10]

Low levels of adiponectin may also promote the inception and progression of various malignancies. Reduced adiponectin can enhance cell proliferation by regulating fibrinogen and CRP as well as induce the production of inflammatory cytokines, such as IL-6 and TNF-α.[11]

Leptin

Leptin, another product of adipocytes, is also a central mediator of inflammation in obesity. Structurally, it is similar to cytokines such as IL-6 and can regulate T cell proliferation and activation. Leptin can also recruit and activate monocytes and macrophages and promote angiogenesis.[12–14] Best known for its effect on appetite regulation, leptin is also associated with asthma, fertility, and other conditions described in more detail.

Insulin Resistance

Insulin resistance occurs with the development of visceral adipose tissue. Normally, the subcutaneous adipose tissue is able to act as a protective metabolic clearinghouse for storage of extra energy that is derived from dietary triglycerides. When the subcutaneous fat is no longer able to perform this function, fat deposition occurs in visceral adipose depots as well as ectopic sites, such as skeletal muscle and liver.[7]

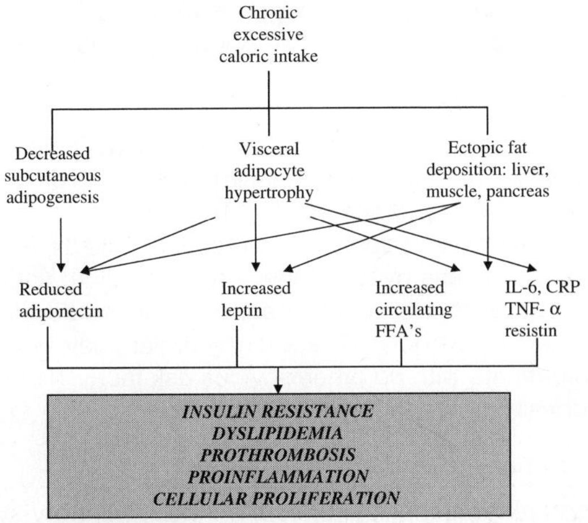

Fig. 1. Pathophysiology of adiposity.

With ectopic adipocyte development, oxidation of fatty acids become defective, and FFAs are allowed to circulate freely in these organs. The excess circulating FFAs result in dyslipidemia and insulin resistance.[8] Insulin resistance with progression to metabolic syndrome, diabetes, and polycystic ovarian syndrome is discussed in detail in a separate article of this series.

Proinflammatory and Prothrombotic Mediation

Markers of a proinflammatory state include elevation of levels of CRP, IL-6, and plasminogen activator inhibitor-1 (PAI-1). IL-6 is secreted by macrophages and T cells and regulated by leptin and adiponectin. Systemic circulation of IL-6 is thought to be involved in both the pathogenesis and progression of asthma, sleep apnea, malignancies, metabolic syndrome, and cardiovascular disease.[11,15–17]

CLINICAL MANIFESTATIONS OF OBESITY

Cardiovascular Disease

Through the mechanisms of hyperglycemia, prothrombotic state, proinflammatory mediation, elevated blood pressure, and atherogenic dyslipidemia, visceral obesity increases the risk of cardiovascular disease.[16,18] This clustering of risk factors is clinically known as metabolic syndrome or insulin resistance syndrome. Metabolic syndrome is discussed in detail in a separate article.

The triad of the atherogenic process—atherosclerosis, inflammation, and thrombosis—is modulated by insulin resistance and adipokines.[19] Increased exposure of hepatocytes to FFAs by inadequate adipocyte fatty acid oxidation promotes dyslipidemia.[8] When circulating FFAs, especially LDL, are higher, the atherosclerotic plaque, which is rich in lipids and macrophages, enlarges. Atherosclerotic plaque development is accelerated by low levels of HDL, elevated blood pressure, inflammatory cytokines, and elevated plasma glucose levels, all of which are mediated by insulin resistance and elevated FFA circulation.

Visceral adiposity affects not only plaque development but, more importantly, also plaque disruption. When the advanced atherosclerotic plaque becomes unstable, it can rupture and cause an acute coronary syndrome. This rupture in a milieu of already prothrombotic state of insulin resistance can promote propagation of thrombi, which can worsen further syndromes.[19] Mechanisms in all stages of plaque formation, rupture and thrombosis, may be influenced by adiponectin. Adiponectin linked with the inflammatory markers CRP and fibrinogen is also positively correlated with HDL cholesterol, negatively correlated with apolipoprotein B-100, and triacylglyerols.[20]

Cardiac Structure and Obesity

Obesity may be related to remodeling of the structure of the myocardium.[21] However, it is unclear if obesity is the causal mechanism or if comorbid conditions, such as obstructive sleep apnea (OSA), diabetes, and hypertension, are the causal mechanisms.[22] All these conditions, and possibly a direct effect of adiposity mediated by leptin and adiponectin, may cause hypertrophy and heart failure.[23] Cardiac arrhythmias may occur in obese patients, but more often, arrhythmias develop in the setting of OSA or left ventricular hypertrophy. These arrhythmias may increase the likelihood of sudden death in patients with no other obvious risk factor for hypertrophy or heart failure other than obesity.[24]

Respiratory Manifestations of Pathogenic Obesity

Obesity causes important mechanical effects on the respiratory system. Excess soft tissue mass and fatty infiltration of the chest wall and increased pulmonary blood volume cause a decrease in respiratory muscle compliance, functional residual capacity and total volume, and peripheral airway diameter, as well as alterations in pulmonary blood volume and a ventilation-perfusion mismatch.[25,26] Although obesity may also cause an increase in airway hyper-responsiveness, this claim remains controversial.[25,27–29]

Obstructive Sleep Apnea

OSA is characterized by repetitive upper airway collapse during sleep, which causes hypoxia, sympathetic nervous system surges, airway edema, and inflammation.[17] The intermittent airflow obstruction triggers increases in local and systemic inflammatory markers and oxidative stress. These levels of proinflammatory cytokines, such as IL-6, TNF-α, and leptin, and reduced adiponectin levels are comparable to those of obese patients, suggesting that obesity may mediate these responses, both in cause and in effect.[17,30] A vicious cycle can worsen in which significant changes in sleep patterns during OSA can promote weight gain by modulating appetite-regulating hormones.[31]

Shore[30] suggests that OSA may be in the causal pathway between obesity and the development of asthma. With the persistent state of enhanced vagal tone and constant upper airway obstruction, local and systemic inflammation occurs. These inflammatory changes cause changes in intrathoracic pressure, which in turn causes bronchoconstriction and gastroesophageal reflux. Moreover, cytokine production and oxidative stress may trigger bronchial hyperreactivity.

Asthma

Cross-sectional studies have shown an increased prevalence of asthma in the obese.[32] In addition, some controlled prospective cohort studies noted a dose-response relationship with incident asthma and BMI.[33,34] One cross-sectional study found that obese adults with insulin resistance had an increased risk of aeroallergen sensitization, specifically increased immunoglobulin E antibodies to common inhalant allergens, and allergic, but not nonallergic, asthma.[35] Gastroesophageal reflux disease (GERD) and sleep-disordered breathing are 2 conditions commonly associated with obesity and asthma, but they are independently related.[36] Both obesity and OSA exacerbate symptoms of asthma.[37] Obesity may affect a patient's atopic status, but this relationship remains controversial.[37]

Although biological mechanisms between obesity and asthma have not yet been fully elucidated, a strongly suspected contributor is leptin, which stimulates elevated levels of eotaxin (an eosinophil chemoattractant), and alterations in lung volume.[38] Studies in animal models suggest that leptin appears to have an important immunomodulatory role that may affect airway function and immune response.[30,39] Leptin also, however, affects normal lung development, specifically by mediating pulmonary surfactant synthesis and the differentiation of lipofibroblasts into mature normal fibroblasts in the lung.[38,40]

Gastrointestinal Manifestations of Pathogenic Obesity

Gastroesophageal reflux disease

GERD affects 20% of the US population and more than 30% of obese patients and has a linear relationship to BMI.[41] Abdominal obesity, more than obesity alone, may be related to GERD development.[42]

As described here, GERD is associated with the risk of asthma in obese individuals.[36] Moreover, obese individuals with GERD are more likely to have other complications, including erosive GERD. Obesity is a significant risk factor for the development of a hiatal hernia, which in turn increases the risk of lower esophageal sphincter (LES) displacement and reduction of LES tone, both of which exacerbate esophagitis.[43] However, obesity appears to have only an indirect increased risk of developing Barrett esophagus, through the precursor lesion of GERD.[43,44] Visceral adipokines, such as leptin, IL-6, and TNF-α, may stimulate progression into Barrett esophagus and possibly esophageal adenocarcinoma.[43]

Nonalcoholic Fatty Liver Disease and Steatohepatitis

Nonalcoholic Fatty Liver Disease (NAFLD) is considered the hepatic manifestation of the insulin resistance syndrome.[45] Triglyceride accumulation within the liver is the primary feature of NAFLD, but it can also lead to recruitment of inflammatory cells and fibrosis. About one-third of the US population may have NAFLD.[45] Far from being benign, NAFLD is the leading cause of chronic liver disease in the United States, and those with NAFLD have a higher mortality rate than that of age-, gender-, and BMI-matched controls. Patients with NAFLD have a 5%, 7-year risk of developing cirrhosis.[46]

NAFLD is associated with obesity, primarily central adiposity, leading to insulin resistance.[45] Due to impairments of fatty acid oxidation and increased lipolysis during insulin resistance, triglyceride accumulation occurs as ectopic fat depots in the liver. Moreover, hyperinsulinemia promotes more hepatic triglyceride and FFA production. The FFAs travel between adipocytes and hepatocytes and bring adiponectin and TNF-α.[10] TNF-α antagonizes adiponectin to promote steatosis and insulin resistance.[9]

It is postulated that cirrhosis develops when this unopposed, or poorly opposed, TNF-α causes oxidant stress and high levels of inflammatory mediators within the liver, cell death, and insulin resistance. These conditions cause activation of hepatic stellate cells to repair cells. These cells are modulated by leptin, adiponectin, angiotensin, and norepinephrine. Moreover, when the liver is unable to adequately repair the hepatocytes, cirrhosis develops.[47]

The mainstay of management of NAFLD is diet and exercise, leading to slow weight reduction, as rapid weight loss can worsen inflammation.[48] Insulin-sensitizing agents, such as metformin and particularly thiazolidinediones, because of the inhibitory effect of peroxisome proliferator-activated receptor agonists on inflammation, have reduced symptoms of NAFLD.[49,50] However, lipid-lowering agents have no proven benefit.[45]

Gallstone Disease

Three factors promote the development of gallstones: gallbladder hypomotility, bile supersaturation with cholesterol, and bile destabilization by kinetic protein factors.[51] In obese patients, cholesterol hypersecretion and supersaturation increase the uptake or synthesis of cholesterol from within the liver, resulting in increased biliary cholesterol secretion. Gallbladder emptying in response to cholecystokinin or a meal is impaired in patients with gallstones.[52] Gallstone formation is strongly related to abdominal adiposity, hyperinsulinemia, and dyslipidemia but only in those with a genetic predisposition to gallstone formation.[53,54] Abdominally obese patients and those with elevations in FFAs and insulin resistance have persistently increased cholesterol synthesis, the primary link. Leptin may also increase the susceptibility of obese patients to gallstone development. Some, but not all, studies suggest that leptin has been found to modulate genes that regulate cholesterol gallstone synthesis.[55,56]

Obese patients undergoing gastric bypass or banding appear to have an even greater increased risk of gallstone formation. In this circumstance, bile stasis is the more likely mechanism responsible for rapid weight loss.[51,57] Some researchers have considered routine screening for gallstone disease before surgery; however, several studies show that ultrasound screening in the absence of symptoms before surgery is not indicated. Those who have symptoms should be screened and have prophylactic cholecystectomy. Those who have intraoperative evidence of gallstones may also warrant preventive surgery.[57,58]

Malignancy

Several malignancies are thought to be related to obesity. The major candidates relating obesity to cancer are those cytokines that cause insulin resistance: leptin, IL-6, TNF-α, adiponectin, and FFAs.[4,59] These cytokines are involved in the promotion of cellular proliferation and in the inhibition of apoptosis.[60] Adiponectin, the most abundant hormone secreted by adipocytes, is likely a key protector and regulator in cell proliferation in this process, both by acting directly on cancer cells and indirectly through the pathway of insulin resistance.[11] Insulin resistance and hyperinsulinemia promote the production of insulin-like growth factor-I (IGF-1). Many cancer cell lines, including prostate, breast, and colon, have IGF-1 receptors.[61] Additionally, visceral adipocytes, by way of lipolysis, increase the circulating level of FFAs.[59] FFAs may have cancer potential both directly, by causing cellular proliferation, and indirectly, through insulin resistance.[59] FFAs and other cytokines recruit the sympathetic nervous system and cause cell proliferation, by directly stimulating IGF-1 as well as other growth factors, including platelet-derived growth factor-BB, but these relationships are yet to be established.[11]

Adiponectin receptors are also expressed in several cancer cell types, including prostate, hepatocellular, breast, endometrial, colonic, and neuroblastoma cancer cell lines, and may suppress cell growth. Low levels of adiponectin are also associated with renal cell cancer, gastric cancer, and leukemia after controlling for BMI but was not considered significant after controlling for waist-to-hip ratio (WHR).[11]

Circulating concentrations of adiponectin are reduced in obesity and most closely correlate with markers of insulin sensitivity.[62] High adiponectin concentrations may also be correlated with reduced inflammation by reducing the growth of macrophages and adhesion molecules, but the mechanisms are still being defined.[11]

Breast Cancer

Obesity has a complex relationship with breast cancer risk, progression, remission, and recurrence. In a review by Althuis and colleagues, only postmenopausal women seemed to have a consistent association of obesity with hormone-receptor-positive breast cancer.[63] In studies regarding women with postmenopausal breast cancer when circulating estrogen levels are low, low levels of adiponectin were associated with an increased cancer risk, independent of BMI, leptin levels, or IGF-1.[62,64] Some large cohort studies showed that the presence of obesity or overweight before diagnosis was associated with increased risk of recurrence and death from all types of breast cancer.[65,66] Some data suggest that the etiology of poor outcomes is that obese women have higher circulating levels of tumor-promoting estrogen and testosterone as well as reduced cellular immunity.[67] However, other studies failed to find a correlation.[68,69]

Endometrial Cancer

Endometrial cancer has long been known to be associated with obesity and distribution of adipose tissue.[70,71] The risk is greater in obese women with associated hypertension, diabetes, or polycystic ovarian syndrome.[72] The putative mechanisms for development are, as in breast cancer, higher circulating levels of unopposed ɪn and ovarian hyperandrogenism, causing elevated levels of testosterone, ssibly hypersecretion of leutinizing hormone.[73,74] Endometrial cancer is also associated with low levels of adiponectin, with a risk 6.5 times that of obese women with higher circulating adiponectin levels.[75]

Colon and Rectal Cancer

The association of obesity with colorectal cancer varies by gender. An increased risk of colon cancer is noted in men but the relationship for women is weak and inconsistent. In a meta-analysis performed by Larsson and Wolk, the relative risk of colon and rectal cancer was shown in men but not in women. Risk increased with increasing waist circumference and WHR, suggesting that visceral adipose tissue may be more closely associated.[76] One large prospective, nested case control study revealed that men with the highest levels of adiponectin had a 60% reduced risk of colon cancer, even after adjusting for body size, waist circumference, and physical activity.[77] Hypertriglyceridemia, hyperinsulinemia, and the development of IGF-1 have also been shown to be associated with elevated risk of colorectal cancer, especially in adenomas.[60] Long-term chronic inflammation of the colonic tissue also creates carcinogenesis and may be mediated by adipose tissue inflammatory cytokines, including IL-6, TNF-α, and adiponectin.[43]

Prostate Cancer

Screening for prostate cancer is difficult in obese men. Prostate-specific antigen levels are inversely related to BMI, possibly due to increased plasma volume levels in obese men.[78] According to studies by Wright and colleagues and Gong and colleagues,[79,80] the incidence of prostate cancer is not significantly elevated for obese men. Unfortunately, for those men who do develop prostate cancer, progression to later stages and mortality are increased in those who are obese. Prostate cancer was also found to be associated with lower levels of adiponectin and high adipokine concentrations of leptin, IL-6, and vascular endothelial growth factor.[81,82] Once prostate cancer has developed, obesity appears to increase the risk of aggressive cancer, but it may be protective for individuals with nonaggressive cancer.[83]

Renal Cell Carcinoma

In reviews by Lipworth and colleagues and Calle and Kaaks,[84,85] obesity was found to be associated with 30% of renal cell adenocarcinomas. It is suspected that the mechanism for cancer induction may be lipid peroxidation, which is common in obese patients. Moreover, elevations in IGF-1 and high glomerular infiltration rates, independent of hypertension, may also contribute.

Other Cancers

Other malignancies may be associated with obesity, but the relationships remain controversial or exploratory thus far. Adiponectin may also be associated with other malignancies, including gastric cancer and acute myeloblastic leukemia.[11] The evidence for an effect of obesity on epithelial ovarian cancer has been inconclusive; however, a meta-analysis by Olsen and colleagues[86] suggests that obesity confers a 1.3 risk of ovarian cancer. An indirect elevated risk for esophageal adenocarcinoma, by way of Barrett esophagus, may also occur.[43,44] Evidence also suggests a relationship between obesity and diabetes to pancreatic cancer, but the mechanisms remain speculative.[83]

Despite the associations of obesity with several cancers, no specific recommendations exist to target obese persons for cancer screening. Unfortunately, obese women are less likely to seek preventive health care screening or receive preventative cancer screening. Targeted screening may be warranted for specific cancers, such as breast and cervical cancer.[87]

SKIN MANIFESTATIONS OF OBESITY

Obesity causes abnormalities in several functions of the skin, including in the effects on the sebaceous gland, sebum production, skin barrier function, and sweat production. It also promotes changes in lymphatics, collagen structure and function, wound healing, and subcutaneous fat.[88] Two gene products are thought to mediate these skin abnormalities in obese patients, leptin and pro-opiomelanocortin.[88] Some of the major problems with the skin are listed briefly.

The major metabolic manifestations of skin disorders in obese individuals are modulated through insulin resistance. Obesity worsens the severity of acne through hyperandrogenism and increased production of IGF-1, which activate sebaceous glands.[89] Other conditions mediated by insulin resistance are keratosis pilaris, acanthosis nigricans, hirsutism, and acrochordons.[88]

Skin problems are also caused by mechanical means and among them are chronic venous insufficiency, lymphedema, striae, cellulite development, and adiposis dolorosa (painful multiple subcutaneous lipomas). Lymphedema and venous stasis can lead to a chronic inflammatory state. Patients with these conditions are more prone to cellulitis, panniculitis, venous stasis ulcers, necrotizing fasciitis, and possibly even angiosarcoma.[88]

Hidradenitis suppurativa, caused by chronic recurrent infections of the apocrine glands, may be exacerbated by obesity.[90] Finally, a higher prevalence of psoriasis exists in obese compared with that in normal-weight patients. The long-term prognosis of psoriasis worsens with increasing BMI.[91]

MUSCULOSKELETAL DISABILITY AND PAIN ASSOCIATED WITH OBESITY

Obesity can cause several effects on musculoskeletal function. Adiposity is positively related to musculoskeletal pain and injury, especially in the back, hip, knee, ankle, and foot.[92] Biomechanical adaptations caused by the sheer bulk and force of increased fat mass affect locomotion, balance, and strength and cause pain. Obese individuals have an altered center of gravity, and some inertia is apparent due to increased anteroposterior sway. Postural control and balance may be intact and is quite dependent on physical activity. The energy cost of walking incurred is greater as weight rises, but whether the inefficiency is due to physiologic or mechanical origins, or both, is unclear.[93] The obese gait can be differentiated from normal gaits by greater hip abduction, reduced hip flexion, and reduced ankle plantar flexion. These adjustments may have an impact on the development of maladaptations. Obesity may have a profound effect not only on joints but also the tendons, fascia, and cartilage. These adjustments are made to reduce the load on the knee joint.[94]

Osteoarthritis

Osteoarthritis (OA) is a degenerative joint disorder in which obesity has an increased risk of incidence and progression in weight-bearing joints.[92,95] Although there may be some metabolic factors increasing the risk of OA in obesity, the primary etiology tends to be persistent loading during joint movement and locomotion.[96]

In the knee, obese patients have an increased load on the medial compartment due to varus joint malalignment. Although the load is increased, no parallel increase in subchondral cartilage volume occurs to support this load.[92] Muscular strength and mass may be more important than adiposity or cartilage volume in its development. Muscles in fatigue are less able to attenuate the shock of a load on the joint. Obese individuals have greater absolute but lesser relative muscle strength, thus muscle strengthening and physical activity can reduce the disability and pain associated with knee OA.[92,93,95]

Plantar Fasciitis

Obese individuals have a 5-fold greater risk of developing plantar fasciitis than nonobese individuals. Research of obese individuals has shown that plantar pressures correlate moderately with body weight, with higher pressures under the heel, midfoot, and central metatarsal heads during walking. This relationship is particularly strong in obese women, who may have weaker ligaments in the medial longitudinal arch than those of men.[97] The relationship of plantar pressure to the development of heel pain, however, is unclear. Research has implicated arch function, compressibility of the plantar fat pad, and elevated plantar pressures in pain development, but the ultimate link remains controversial.[92]

SUMMARY

Obesity, especially visceral adiposity, appears to be associated with several clinical conditions and can cause profound disease and disability. Adipocyte regulatory adipokines may be responsible for disease promotion and progression in several of these conditions. The sheer bulk of mass, weight, and displacement exacerbates others. Further studies will be needed to truly solidify these connections and to make them indisputable. Indeed Bays and colleagues[2] propose labeling the metabolic dysregulation caused by adipocytes "adiposopathy." Once these relationships are solidified, more specific treatment targets can be identified at earlier stages, thus preventing progression of pathogenic adiposity to disease.

REFERENCES

1. Bays H, Blonde L, Rosenson R. Adiposopathy: how do diet, exercise and weight loss drug therapies improve metabolic disease in overweight patients? Expert Rev Cardiovasc Ther 2006;4(6):871–95.
2. Bays HE, Gonzalez-Campoy JM, Bray GA, et al. Pathogenic potential of adipose tissue and metabolic consequences of adipocyte hypertrophy and increased visceral adiposity. Expert Rev Cardiovasc Ther 2008;6(3):343–68.
3. Hamilton MT, Hamilton DG, Zderic TW. Role of low energy expenditure and sitting in obesity, metabolic syndrome, type 2 diabetes, and cardiovascular disease. Diabetes 2007;56(11):2655–67.
4. Ronti T, Lupattelli G, Mannarino E. The endocrine function of adipose tissue: an update. Clin Endocrinol (Oxf) 2006;64(4):355–65.
5. de Ferranti S, Mozaffarian D. The perfect storm: obesity, adipocyte dysfunction, and metabolic consequences. Clin Chem 2008;54(6):945–55.
6. Redinger RN. The physiology of adiposity. J Ky Med Assoc 2008;106(2):53–62.
7. Despres JP, Lemieux I, Bergeron J, et al. Abdominal obesity and the metabolic syndrome: contribution to global cardiometabolic risk. Arterioscler Thromb Vasc Biol 2008;28(6):1039–49.

8. Rader DJ. Effect of insulin resistance, dyslipidemia, and intra-abdominal adiposity on the development of cardiovascular disease and diabetes mellitus. Am J Med 2007;120(Suppl 1):S12–8.
9. Arner P. The adipocyte in insulin resistance: key molecules and the impact of the thiazolidinediones. Trends Endocrinol Metab 2003;14(3):137–45.
10. Whitehead JP, Richards AA, Hickman IJ, et al. Adiponectin–a key adipokine in the metabolic syndrome. Diabetes Obes Metab 2006;8(3):264–80.
11. Barb D, Williams CJ, Neuwirth AK, et al. Adiponectin in relation to malignancies: a review of existing basic research and clinical evidence. Am J Clin Nutr 2007; 86(3):s858–66.
12. Sierra-Honigmann MR, Nath AK, Murakami C, et al. Biological action of leptin as an angiogenic factor. Science 1998;281(5383):1683–6.
13. Wellen KE, Hotamisligil GS. Obesity-induced inflammatory changes in adipose tissue. J Clin Invest 2003;112(12):1785–8.
14. Weyer C, Foley JE, Bogardus C, et al. Enlarged subcutaneous abdominal adipocyte size, but not obesity itself, predicts type II diabetes independent of insulin resistance. Diabetologia 2000;43(12):1498–506.
15. Bahrami H, Bluemke DA, Kronmal R, et al. Novel metabolic risk factors for incident heart failure and their relationship with obesity: the MESA (Multi-Ethnic Study of Atherosclerosis) study. J Am Coll Cardiol 2008;51(18):1775–83.
16. Despres JP. Cardiovascular disease under the influence of excess visceral fat. Crit Pathw Cardiol 2007;6(2):51–9.
17. Mehra R, Redline S. Sleep apnea: a proinflammatory disorder that coaggregates with obesity. J Allergy Clin Immunol 2008;121(5):1096–102.
18. Grundy SM. Metabolic syndrome pandemic. Arterioscler Thromb Vasc Biol 2008; 28(4):629–36.
19. Corti R, Hutter R, Badimon JJ, et al. Evolving concepts in the triad of atherosclerosis, inflammation and thrombosis. J Thromb Thrombolysis 2004;17(1):35–44.
20. Schulze MB, Rimm EB, Shai I, et al. Relationship between adiponectin and glycemic control, blood lipids, and inflammatory markers in men with type 2 diabetes. Diabetes Care 2004;27(7):1680–7.
21. Abel ED, Litwin SE, Sweeney G. Cardiac remodeling in obesity. Physiol Rev 2008; 88(2):389–419.
22. Owan T, Litwin SE. Is there a cardiomyopathy of obesity? Curr Heart Fail Rep 2007;4(4):221–8.
23. Alpert MA, Fraley MA, Birchem JA, et al. Management of obesity cardiomyopathy. Expert Rev Cardiovasc Ther 2005;3(2):225–30.
24. Fraley MA, Birchem JA, Senkottaiyan N, et al. Obesity and the electrocardiogram. Obes Rev 2005;6(4):275–81.
25. Chinn S, Jarvis D, Burney P. Relation of bronchial responsiveness to body mass index in the ECRHS. European Community Respiratory Health Survey. Thorax 2002;57(12):1028–33.
26. Weiner P, Waizman J, Weiner M, et al. Influence of excessive weight loss after gastroplasty for morbid obesity on respiratory muscle performance. Thorax 1998;53(1):39–42.
27. Bibi H, Shoseyov D, Feigenbaum D, et al. The relationship between asthma and obesity in children: is it real or a case of over diagnosis? J Asthma 2004;41(4): 403–10.
28. Litonjua AA, Sparrow D, Celedon JC, et al. Association of body mass index with the development of methacholine airway hyperresponsiveness in men: the Normative Aging Study. Thorax 2002;57(7):581–5.

29. Schachter LM, Salome CM, Peat JK, et al. Obesity is a risk for asthma and wheeze but not airway hyperresponsiveness. Thorax 2001;56(1):4–8.
30. Shore SA. Obesity and asthma: possible mechanisms. J Allergy Clin Immunol 2008;121(5):1087–93.
31. Patel SR, Malhotra A, White DP, et al. Association between reduced sleep and weight gain in women. Am J Epidemiol 2006;164(10):947–54.
32. Ford ES. The epidemiology of obesity and asthma. J Allergy Clin Immunol 2005; 115(5):897–909.
33. Ford ES, Mannino DM, Redd SC, et al. Body mass index and asthma incidence among USA adults. Eur Respir J 2004;24(5):740–4.
34. Nystad W, Meyer HE, Nafstad P, et al. Body mass index in relation to adult asthma among 135,000 Norwegian men and women. Am J Epidemiol 2004;160(10): 969–76.
35. Husemoen LL, Glumer C, Lau C, et al. Association of obesity and insulin resistance with asthma and aeroallergen sensitization. Allergy 2008;63(5):575–82.
36. Gunnbjornsdottir MI, Omenaas E, Gislason T, et al. Obesity and nocturnal gastro-oesophageal reflux are related to onset of asthma and respiratory symptoms. Eur Respir J 2004;24(1):116–21.
37. Kasasbeh A, Kasasbeh E, Krishnaswamy G. Potential mechanisms connecting asthma, esophageal reflux, and obesity/sleep apnea complex–a hypothetical review. Sleep Med Rev 2007;11(1):47–58.
38. Beuther DA, Weiss ST, Sutherland ER. Obesity and asthma. Am J Respir Crit Care Med 2006;174(2):112–9.
39. Mito N, Kitada C, Hosoda T, et al. Effect of diet-induced obesity on ovalbumin-specific immune response in a murine asthma model. Metabolism 2002;51(10): 1241–6.
40. Mancuso P, Huffnagle GB, Olszewski MA, et al. Leptin corrects host defense defects after acute starvation in murine pneumococcal pneumonia. Am J Respir Crit Care Med 2006;173(2):212–8.
41. Flegal KM, Carroll MD, Ogden CL, et al. Prevalence and trends in obesity among US adults, 1999-2000. JAMA 2002;288(14):1723–7.
42. El-Serag HB, Ergun GA, Pandolfino J, et al. Obesity increases oesophageal acid exposure. Gut 2007;56(6):749–55.
43. Watanabe S, Hojo M, Nagahara A. Metabolic syndrome and gastrointestinal diseases. J Gastroenterol 2007;42(4):267–74.
44. Cook MB, Greenwood DC, Hardie LJ, et al. A systematic review and meta-analysis of the risk of increasing adiposity on Barrett's esophagus. Am J Gastroenterol 2008;103(2):292–300.
45. Abdelmalek MF, Diehl AM. Nonalcoholic fatty liver disease as a complication of insulin resistance. Med Clin North Am 2007;91(6):1125–49.
46. Adams LA, Lymp JF, St Sauver J, et al. The natural history of nonalcoholic fatty liver disease: a population-based cohort study. Gastroenterology 2005;129(1): 113–21.
47. Bataller R, Brenner DA. Liver fibrosis. J Clin Invest 2005;115(2):209–18.
48. Andersen T, Gluud C, Franzmann MB, et al. Hepatic effects of dietary weight loss in morbidly obese subjects. J Hepatol 1991;12(2):224–9.
49. Schreuder TC, Verwer BJ, van Nieuwkerk CM, et al. Nonalcoholic fatty liver disease: An overview of current insights in pathogenesis, diagnosis and treatment. World J Gastroenterol 2008;14(16):2474–86.
50. Torres DM, Harrison SA. Diagnosis and therapy of nonalcoholic steatohepatitis. Gastroenterology 2008;134(6):1682–98.

51. Grunhage F, Lammert F. Gallstone disease. Pathogenesis of gallstones: a genetic perspective. Best Pract Res Clin Gastroenterol 2006;20(6):997–1015.
52. Paumgartner G, Sauerbruch T. Gallstones: pathogenesis. Lancet 1991; 338(8775):1117–21.
53. Boland LL, Folsom AR, Rosamond WD. Hyperinsulinemia, dyslipidemia, and obesity as risk factors for hospitalized gallbladder disease. A prospective study. Ann Epidemiol 2002;12(2):131–40.
54. Tsai CJ, Leitzmann MF, Willett WC, et al. Prospective study of abdominal adiposity and gallstone disease in US men. Am J Clin Nutr 2004;80(1):38–44.
55. Graewin SJ, Kiely JM, Lu D, et al. Leptin regulates gallbladder genes related to gallstone pathogenesis in leptin-deficient mice. J Am Coll Surg 2008;206(3): 503–10.
56. Mendez-Sanchez N, Bermejo-Martinez L, Chavez-Tapia NC, et al. Obesity-related leptin receptor polymorphisms and gallstones disease. Ann Hepatol 2006;5(2):97–102.
57. Kiewiet RM, Durian MF, van Leersum M, et al. Gallstone formation after weight loss following gastric banding in morbidly obese Dutch patients. Obes Surg 2006;16(5):592–6.
58. Taylor J, Leitman IM, Horowitz M. Is routine cholecystectomy necessary at the time of Roux-en-Y gastric bypass? Obes Surg 2006;16(6):759–61.
59. Hsu IR, Kim SP, Kabir M, et al. Metabolic syndrome, hyperinsulinemia, and cancer. Am J Clin Nutr 2007;86(3):s867–71.
60. Giovannucci E. Metabolic syndrome, hyperinsulinemia, and colon cancer: a review. Am J Clin Nutr 2007;86(3):s836–42.
61. Pollak M. Insulin-like growth factor-related signaling and cancer development. Recent Results Cancer Res 2007;174:49–53.
62. Tworoger SS, Eliassen AH, Kelesidis T, et al. Plasma adiponectin concentrations and risk of incident breast cancer. J Clin Endocrinol Metab 2007;92(4): 1510–6.
63. Althuis MD, Fergenbaum JH, Garcia-Closas M, et al. Etiology of hormone receptor-defined breast cancer: a systematic review of the literature. Cancer Epidemiol Biomarkers Prev 2004;13(10):1558–68.
64. Mantzoros C, Petridou E, Dessypris N, et al. Adiponectin and breast cancer risk. J Clin Endocrinol Metab 2004;89(3):1102–7.
65. Calle EE, Rodriguez C, Walker-Thurmond K, et al. Overweight, obesity, and mortality from cancer in a prospectively studied cohort of U.S. adults. N Engl J Med 2003;348(17):1625–38.
66. Kroenke CH, Chen WY, Rosner B, et al. Weight, weight gain, and survival after breast cancer diagnosis. J Clin Oncol 2005;23(7):1370–8.
67. Key TJ, Appleby PN, Reeves GK, et al. Body mass index, serum sex hormones, and breast cancer risk in postmenopausal women. J Natl Cancer Inst 2003;95(16): 1218–26.
68. Carmichael AR. Obesity and prognosis of breast cancer. Obes Rev 2006;7(4): 333–40.
69. Carmichael AR. Obesity as a risk factor for development and poor prognosis of breast cancer. BJOG 2006;113(10):1160–6.
70. Levi F, La Vecchia C, Negri E, et al. Body mass at different ages and subsequent endometrial cancer risk. Int J Cancer 1992;50(4):567–71.
71. Swanson CA, Potischman N, Wilbanks GD, et al. Relation of endometrial cancer risk to past and contemporary body size and body fat distribution. Cancer Epidemiol Biomarkers Prev 1993;2(4):321–7.

72. Weiderpass E, Persson I, Adami HO, et al. Body size in different periods of life, diabetes mellitus, hypertension, and risk of postmenopausal endometrial cancer (Sweden). Cancer Causes Control 2000;11(2):185–92.
73. Hardiman P, Pillay OC, Atiomo W. Polycystic ovary syndrome and endometrial carcinoma. Lancet 2003;361(9371):1810–2.
74. Kaaks R, Lukanova A, Kurzer MS. Obesity, endogenous hormones, and endometrial cancer risk: a synthetic review. Cancer Epidemiol Biomarkers Prev 2002; 11(12):1531–43.
75. Dal Maso L, Augustin LS, Karalis A, et al. Circulating adiponectin and endometrial cancer risk. J Clin Endocrinol Metab 2004;89(3):1160–3.
76. Larsson SC, Wolk A. Obesity and colon and rectal cancer risk: a meta-analysis of prospective studies. Am J Clin Nutr 2007;86(3):556–65.
77. Wei EK, Giovannucci E, Fuchs CS, et al. Low plasma adiponectin levels and risk of colorectal cancer in men: a prospective study. J Natl Cancer Inst 2005;97(22): 1688–94.
78. Rundle A, Neugut AI. Obesity and screening PSA levels among men undergoing an annual physical exam. Prostate 2008;68(4):373–80.
79. Gong Z, Agalliu I, Lin DW, et al. Obesity is associated with increased risks of prostate cancer metastasis and death after initial cancer diagnosis in middle-aged men. Cancer 2007;109(6):1192–202.
80. Wright ME, Chang SC, Schatzkin A, et al. Prospective study of adiposity and weight change in relation to prostate cancer incidence and mortality. Cancer 2007;109(4):675–84.
81. Michalakis K, Williams CJ, Mitsiades N, et al. Serum adiponectin concentrations and tissue expression of adiponectin receptors are reduced in patients with prostate cancer: a case control study. Cancer Epidemiol Biomarkers Prev 2007;16(2): 308–13.
82. Mistry T, Digby JE, Desai KM, et al. Obesity and prostate cancer: a role for adipokines. Eur Urol 2007;52(1):46–53.
83. Giovannucci E, Michaud D. The role of obesity and related metabolic disturbances in cancers of the colon, prostate, and pancreas. Gastroenterology 2007;132(6):2208–25.
84. Calle EE, Kaaks R. Overweight, obesity and cancer: epidemiological evidence and proposed mechanisms. Nat Rev Cancer 2004;4(8):579–91.
85. Lipworth L, Tarone RE, McLaughlin JK. The epidemiology of renal cell carcinoma. J Urol 2006;176(6):2353–8.
86. Olsen CM, Green AC, Whiteman DC, et al. Obesity and the risk of epithelial ovarian cancer: a systematic review and meta-analysis. Eur J Cancer 2007; 43(4):690–709.
87. Cohen SS, Palmieri RT, Nyante SJ, et al. Obesity and screening for breast, cervical, and colorectal cancer in women: a review. Cancer 2008;112(9): 1892–904.
88. Yosipovitch G, DeVore A, Dawn A. Obesity and the skin: skin physiology and skin manifestations of obesity. J Am Acad Dermatol 2007;56(6):901–16.
89. Cappel M, Mauger D, Thiboutot D. Correlation between serum levels of insulin-like growth factor 1, dehydroepiandrosterone sulfate, and dihydrotestosterone and acne lesion counts in adult women. Arch Dermatol 2005;141(3):333–8.
90. Slade DE, Powell BW, Mortimer PS. Hidradenitis suppurativa: pathogenesis and management. Br J Plast Surg 2003;56(5):451–61.
91. Sakai R, Matsui S, Fukushima M, et al. Prognostic factor analysis for plaque psoriasis. Dermatology 2005;211(2):103–6.

92. Wearing SC, Hennig EM, Byrne NM, et al. Musculoskeletal disorders associated with obesity: a biomechanical perspective. Obes Rev 2006;7(3):239–50.
93. Wearing SC, Hennig EM, Byrne NM, et al. The biomechanics of restricted movement in adult obesity. Obes Rev 2006;7(1):13–24.
94. Spyropoulos P, Pisciotta JC, Pavlou KN, et al. Biomechanical gait analysis in obese men. Arch Phys Med Rehabil 1991;72(13):1065–70.
95. Sarzi-Puttini P, Cimmino MA, Scarpa R, et al. Osteoarthritis: an overview of the disease and its treatment strategies. Semin Arthritis Rheum 2005;35(Suppl 1): 1–10.
96. Powell A, Teichtahl AJ, Wluka AE, et al. Obesity: a preventable risk factor for large joint osteoarthritis which may act through biomechanical factors. Br J Sports Med 2005;39(1):4–5.
97. Hills AP, Hennig EM, McDonald M, et al. Plantar pressure differences between obese and non-obese adults: a biomechanical analysis. Int J Obes Relat Metab Disord 2001;25(11):1674–9.

Obesity and Mental Health

Mary R. Talen, PhD[a,*], Misty M. Mann, MA[b]

KEYWORDS

- Mental health • Obesity • Binge eating disorder
- Behavioral interventions • Body image

In the past 20 years, obesity rates have risen at an alarming rate in children, adolescents, and adults.[1] These changes have spurred initiatives to prevent the long-term physical consequences of obesity on health. However, psychosocial factors and the psychological and emotional functional ability of obese patients also contribute to obesity and weight loss. Limited knowledge exists on the dynamic relationships between mental health and obesity. The assumption is made that obesity creates a psychological burden for people but with little understanding or evidence to support these cultural health beliefs.[2] This article delves into the relationship of mental health and obesity across the lifespan, the effect of obesity treatment on psychosocial functioning, and treatment models that have an effect on patients' mental functioning in the primary care setting.

OBESE CHILDREN AND ADOLESCENTS AND MENTAL HEALTH FUNCTIONING

A common cultural myth states that obese children face more social stressors (eg, teasing, poor peer relationships), poor self-image, and depression than do normal-weight children. In obesity and mental health studies, the psychological functioning of children is largely linked with risk factors in 4 areas: body image, self-esteem, depression, and family functioning.

Body-Image Satisfaction

The more obese children are, the more children and adolescents, particularly girls, report body-image dissatisfaction.[2] Although overweight children and adolescents have lower body-image satisfaction, their dissatisfaction is not significantly higher than that of normal-weight children. "Body dissatisfaction is not, therefore, a unique marker in obesity."[2] Instead, body dissatisfaction is equally evident among normal

[a] Behavioral Health Science, MacNeal Family Medicine Residency Program, 3231 South Euclid Avenue, Berwyn, IL 60402, USA
[b] Argosy University, Chicago, (Formerly the Illinois School of Professional Psychology), 205 North Michigan Avenue, Chicago, IL 60601, USA
* Corresponding author.
E-mail address: mtalen@macneal.com (M.R. Talen).

Prim Care Clin Office Pract 36 (2009) 287–305
doi:10.1016/j.pop.2009.01.012
0095-4543/09/$ – see front matter. Published by Elsevier Inc.
primarycare.theclinics.com

and underweight children. When comparing by cultural and racial differences, obese Hispanic and African American girls follow the same trends as Caucasian girls, with the exception of African American girls with higher body mass indexes (BMI) having higher body satisfaction ratings than those of Hispanic girls.[3,4] In addition, the self-perception of "feeling fat" is a higher risk for emotional problems than the actual weight status.[5] Caucasian and Asian adolescents in particular, who perceive themselves as overweight regardless of their actual weight status, are at increased risk for depression and low self-esteem.[2,5] Project EAT (Eating Among Teens) found that half of teenage girls and a fourth of teenage boys report body dissatisfaction, whereas half of teenage girls and a third of teenage boys use unhealthy weight control methods, such as overly restrictive and binge eating patterns, dieting at an early age, and uncontrolled, disinhibited eating patterns.[6]

Self-Esteem

Another popular health belief—that children and adolescents with low self-esteem tend to be obese and vice versa—is false. The correlation between self-esteem and obesity is modest at best, with many studies reporting children and adolescents having normal ranges of self-esteem.[2,7] Cohort studies of children have identified only modest differences in self-esteem between obese and normal-weight children.[2] In African American children, several studies have found no relationship between BMI and global self-worth.[8] Cultural health beliefs and role models may be contributing factors in self-esteem and body weight. However, in prospective studies with children ranging in age from 5 to 14 years, obese children develop lower self-concepts over time, and children with lower self-esteem become obese.[9] Adolescents are particularly vulnerable to developing poor self-esteem and body image, because self-esteem and body image are rapidly developing during this time. Body image and self-esteem are often influenced by peers, parents, and media.[10] With the stigma surrounding obesity and the media's presentation of an ideal body image, it is no wonder that many adolescent girls, both normal and overweight, express a fear of fat. Moreover, girls as young as those in third grade have engaged in dieting behaviors, and almost 70% of adolescent girls have tried dieting to lose weight.[11] Unhealthy weight control habits, such as early dieting and restrictive eating, along with "feeling fat" may be the precursors to weight gain, poor self-esteem, and possibly BEDs.

Gender and cultural differences may affect a young person's level of self-esteem. Obese girls have lower self-concepts than those of obese boys, and overweight adolescent girls are at greater risk for developing lower self-esteem than overweight boys.[6] When comparing cultural differences, obese Hispanic and Caucasian girls have lower self-esteem, whereas obese African American girls do not report lower self-concepts.[2] Another study of 5- to 10-year-old African American girls has similar results, with no relationship between weight status and global self-worth.[8] Consequently, cultural-social values may play a greater role in the impact of mental health than obesity itself.

Emotions, Mood, and Psychosocial Functioning

Another common belief, not grounded in research, is that depression causes obesity or vice versa. Depression is not significantly correlated with obesity, in clinical or community samples of children.[5,12–14] In a handful of studies, chronically obese boys have slightly higher rates of depression, and depression in childhood may be a risk factor for obesity later.[2,15] Overall, the link between depression in childhood and obesity is poorly understood, and in general, little evidence exists that supports any connection between obesity and depression.

However, depression, anxiety, and eating disorders need to be clinically and treated in overweight and obese children and adolescents. The presence tion-deficit/hyperactivity disorder (ADHD) is a unique characteristic of obese childr and adolescents. Bulimic behaviors (eg, bingeing or purging) have been identified in adolescents with ADHD.[16] Consequently, regular screening for ADHD in obese adolescents, especially those who engage in bulimic behaviors, may be beneficial and aid in treatment planning.

Family and Social Factors

The social climate, including the family, peer, and cultural and socioeconomic contexts, has an affect on weight. Even though the increase in obesity rates cuts across all ages, gender, and socioeconomic status (SES), several factors are significantly correlated with childhood obesity: (1) single female head of households, (2) minority status, (3) parents with less than 12 years of education, (4) more than 1 child in the home, and (5) family income twice the federal poverty level.[17–19] There appears to be significant overlap between the impact of poverty and other environmental family factors, such as food options and choices, controlling and uncontrolled parenting, lack of access to safe physical activities, and the role modeling of eating habits and activity. For example, parental weights are significant factors related to childhood obesity—if one 1 parent is obese, the child has a 40% risk of developing obesity; if 2 parents are obese, this increases to 80%.[20]

Parents have significant influence on a child's weight in other ways. Family role modeling, such as behavioral eating patterns, family meals, amount of physical and other stimulating activities, and food choices are environmental factors that influence the development of obesity in children.[21,22] Parents and caregivers determine the food choices in the home, shape how children learn to monitor their appetite, and influence the amount of a child's physical activity and sedentary activities (eg, television [TV] viewing, video games, sports). Parenting style and its relationship to a child's weight have been identified as significant factors in children's obesity. Overcontrolling parental behavior around eating interferes with a child's ability to self-regulate his/her eating capabilities.[22] When parents impose strict controls over food, especially with preschool children, it has a reverse effect on the child's propensity for high-fat, energy-dense foods. Rather than responding to their own internal cues about how hungry or satisfied they are, children with overcontrolling food environments learn to respond to external rather than internal cues about eating.[23,24] Parents who encourage their child or adolescent to diet (eg, controlling methods) are actually increasing their child's risk for obesity.

On the other extreme, parents who undercontrol access to high-fat, energy-dense foods and sugar-sweetened drinks are placing their children at risk for obesity. Parental role modeling of eating behaviors (eg, binge, frequent, unstructured) is linked to the weight status of children.[24] Planned, nutritious family meals not eaten in front of the TV help to set healthy role modeling and allow children to maintain normal weight status.[24,25] Physical activity and screen time (TV, texting, video games, and computers) have also been linked to increases in weight among children.[24,25] Studies show that sedentary activities—more technology screen time and fewer outdoor sports or play activities—have an impact on childhood weight.[24,26] Again, the role modeling and support of parents to encourage children's physical activity and limit screen time to less that 2 h/d play a significant role in maintaining healthy weight in children.[24,27,28]

In the peer group setting, overweight and obese children are consistently perceived as the "least desirable" in the social pecking order, which may contribute to depression and body-image dissatisfaction.[29,30] The stigma children experience from being overweight or obese affects emotional development. Overweight or obese individuals have been described as lazy, lying, cheating, sloppy, dirty, ugly, stupid, weak willed, and awkward by individuals as young as 6 years of age up to medical professionals.[11,29] Internalizing these stereotypes affects the child's and adolescent's self-esteem and ties their self-worth and weight together.[11] Cultural beliefs about what constitutes being overweight have a strong impact on mental health status. African Americans have less stigma associated with obesity; therefore, weight status has little impact on depression, self-esteem, and body image.

In summary, children and adolescents have more physical consequences than social-emotional problems from obesity.[2,13]

MENTAL HEALTH TREATMENTS IN OBESE CHILDREN AND ADOLESCENTS

Obesity issues have long-term physical and mental health ramifications for children and adolescents into adulthood.[11] The presence of body-image dissatisfaction, mood disorders, low self-esteem, binge eating, or emotional or other disordered eating behaviors must be addressed and referrals made to mental health specialists if appropriate.

In recent reviews of randomized, control trials on lifestyle intervention in treating childhood obesity, family interventions produced significant treatment effects when compared with those with no treatment.[31,32] Interventions that focus on dietary changes, physical activity, and behavior modifications rather than information alone are effective in weight loss, and these changes are maintained over time. Several studies have shown that family-based interventions with only parents may have the greatest treatment effects.[33,34] Meta-analyses on the prevention of childhood obesity have been less promising, showing no changes in BMIs or preventing obesity compared with control groups when children and parents are provided with behavioral interventions (eg, information, dietary changes, and/or physical activity).[35]

Family interventions benefit not only the child but also parents and other siblings. Intervening at the family level widens the opportunities for making behavioral changes, providing new models of healthy eating and increasing activity level.[22] In addition, coaching parents on the benefits of family meals and on providing healthy and nutritious food choices rather than on "good" and "bad" foods creates a different attitude toward food. Parental praise for choosing healthy foods provides positive reinforcement. Moreover, balancing parental controlling behavior around eating is critical. For example, not requiring the child to finish the plate helps the child to recognize internal cues. Using food as a reward or to soothe emotional distress should be discouraged.[20] Finally, parents should monitor how they are responding to their child's and adolescent's eating behaviors, self-esteem, and body image. Families and communities need to teach that self-worth is not tied to body image or relationship to food.[22]

The current recommendations from the American Academy of Pediatrics (AAP) outline a 4-stage approach to the prevention and treatment of childhood obesity for children aged 2 to 19 years[36] (**Table 1**). They include assessment guidelines and recommendations that all patients receive weight management coaching at least once a year. Children with BMIs greater than the 85th percentile should follow the 4-stage protocol. In this model, Stage I protocol focuses on counseling patients and caregivers in dietary styles (eg, healthy choices, fostering self-regulation), physical activities, and monitoring the child for healthy weight status. Stage 2 is a structured weight management protocol that encourages providers to detail dietary and physical

Table 1
Recommendations for treatment of child and adolescent overweight and obesity: AAP, 2007

Stage	Diet	Activities	Goal	Referral
I. Prevention plus	5 + fruits, veggies Breakfast 5–6 family meals Allow child to self-regulate eating with healthy options	< 2 h screen time 1 h physical activity No TV in bedrooms	Weight maintenance	No improvement in 3–6 mo
II. Structured weight management	Plan for balanced diet, low-energy-dense foods Structured daily meal and snack plans	60 min of active play <1 h screen time Increased monitoring by caregivers, health providers	Decreasing BMI, 1 lb/mo not more than 2 lb/wk to healthy weight	No improvements in 3–6 mo, referral to comprehensive treatment program
III. Comprehensive multidisciplinary protocol	Plan for balanced diet, low-energy-dense foods Structured daily meal and snack plans	60 min of active play <1 h screen time Increased monitoring by caregivers, health providers Involvement of caregivers in treatment planning Structured behavior modification goals and monitoring	Weight loss and maintenance to <85th percentile Decreasing BMI, 1 lb/mo not more than 2 lb/wk to healthy weight	BMI 95th percentile w/no improvement advance to stage V
Stage V: Tertiary care protocol	Structured and monitored environment for dietary changes	Structured and monitored physical activity	Surgery assessment Weight loss not more than 2 lb/wk	—

activities, including family meals, less screen time, and 60 minutes of structured play. If patients show no improvement in their BMI after 6 months, they should be referred to Stage 3: comprehensive multidisciplinary team for an intensive, structured, and well-monitored family intervention. Stage 4 is for patients who need a well-controlled environment, intensive medical intervention, and an obesity multidisciplinary treatment team.

OBESE ADULTS AND MENTAL HEALTH

Popular beliefs about obesity and mental health in adults are similar to those about obese children—obese adults suffer from mental health issues. The focus of research includes several different perspectives of mental health functioning and obesity: (1) body-image satisfaction and self-esteem; (2) emotions, mood, and psychosocial functioning; (3) personality characteristics; (4) BEDs; and (5) the family and social-cultural context.

Body-Image Satisfaction and Self-Esteem

Body-image dissatisfaction and weight/shape concerns are emerging as important factors in the mental health of obese patients. Media, peers, family coaches, and teachers play a significant role in influencing body-image satisfaction and eating disorder symptoms.[10,37] Body-image dissatisfaction and weight/shape concerns in adults have a negative impact on psychosocial functioning and are particularly important for women, because society emphasizes thinness.[38] Overall, the mental health differences between normal-weight and obese adults are few. The most pronounced feature of psychosocial impairment is among obese females who have extreme weight/shape concerns. These distressed obese women unduly evaluate themselves in light of their size and shape.[38,39] Like children and adolescents, the level of dissatisfaction with one's body image is associated with poor mental health and not the actual weight status.

Men tend to have lower levels of body-image dissatisfaction. However, men tend to display more body-image dissatisfaction when identifying and striving toward achieving the masculine gender roles and body type. Sexual orientation for men appears to have a link to body-image dissatisfaction, as well. The literature suggests that gay men have a higher level of body-image dissatisfaction when compared with that of their heterosexual counterparts.[40]

Emotions, Moods, and Psychosocial Functioning

One common assumption, not supported by current research, is that obesity and depression are significantly related. One nationally representative study notes that a significant relationship exists only between depression and severely obese (BMI >40) individuals.[41] This phenomenon holds true in other studies: depression and obesity are not correlated.[42,43]

The relationship between obese adults and quality of life based on physical and mental health functioning is another area of research.[43,44] The US Preventive Service Task Force found results similar to those of other international studies in developed countries: obesity is a stronger predictor of poor physical health but not poor mental health.[41,43,45,46] The mental health quality of life is impaired primarily for adults, both men and women, who are severely obese, BMIs >40.[47] Obesity is significantly more prevalent among psychiatric patients (41% male; 50% female) in mental health systems compared with that in the general population (20% male; 27% female).[48] The relationship between psychiatric populations and obesity is unclear. However, psychotropic medications have been suggested as a factor for the increase in obesity among the psychiatric population. Several psychotropic medications are associated with significant weight gain. In turn, weight gain that leads to obesity can affect the quality of life and may predispose the individual to develop depression, thus adding to the number of individuals in the psychiatric population who are obese.[48]

Personality Characteristics and Eating Patterns

No distinctive personality characteristics identify an "obese personality type" using clinical assessment tools, such as the Minnesota Multiphasic Personality Inventory MMPI.[48] Personality traits tend to influence lifestyle behaviors, though, and obese adults tend to be novelty seeking—curious, impulsive, extravagant, and disorderly—along with exhibiting lower persistence and self-directedness.[49] Emotions such as feeling stressed, overwhelmed, or down drive eating patterns and behaviors. Characteristics of obese adults' emotions and eating patterns tend to fall into several categories: emotional eating, eating to combat boredom, and emotional stress eaters.[50] How these behaviors are associated with mental health functioning of obese patients is complex and poorly understood.

Binge Eating Disorders

BED, a pattern of uncontrolled consumption of large quantities of food, has distinct features in adults that separate them from non-BED adults and those with bulimia nervosa (**Box 1**). Adults with BED eat more calories during binge and nonbinge meals and consume more energy from fat than do those without BED. In addition, adults with BED eat for longer periods of time but eat at the same rate as non-BED adults. Those with BED often feel a loss of control when they begin to binge and feel guilty and distressed because of the binge eating. These characteristics can be used to distinguish binge and nonbinge individuals.[51,52] Body-image concerns, frequency of binges, guilt over binge eating, and other eating disorder symptoms contribute to a negative impact on the level of psychosocial functioning.[38,53]

Obese adults tend to have more binge eating behaviors and relate their self-worth to how satisfied they are with their body shape and self-image. BED is more prevalent

Box 1
Binge eating disorder definition, risk factors, and treatment

Defining BED	Risk factors	Treatment
Consuming large amounts of foods in a short period of time (ie, 2 h), more than what would be considered normal for the average person.	Sociocultural emphasis on thinness	Cognitive-behavioral therapy
Feeling out of control during the binge in relationship to the food	Parenting	Interpersonal therapy
Individual feels distress for engaging in the binge eating behaviors	Childhood experiences	Dialectical-behavioral therapy
	Family history related to eating disorders	
	Family history of being overweight, genetic predisposition	
	Being overweight during childhood and adolescence	

among obese women then that among men and has significant comorbidities with depression, anxiety, negative body image, obsessive-compulsive behaviors, and impulsivity.[52] Body-image concerns, frequency of binges, guilt over binge eating, and other eating disorder symptoms contribute to a negative impact on the level of psychosocial functioning. Of those seeking weight loss treatments, 20% to 30% meet criteria for BED.[54] Binge eaters do worse in treatment and regain weight after treatment.[55]

The risk factors for developing BEDs are similar to those ascribed to anorexia nervosa and bulimia nervosa: sociocultural emphasis on thinness, family history related to eating disorders, and vulnerability to being overweight (eg, family history, genetic predisposition).[52] Moreover, a high score on novelty seeking during a personality assessment is related to binge eating and overeating.[49,56] Being overweight in childhood or adolescence may be a precursor to unhealthy eating patterns and poor weight control habits. In overweight, treatment-seeking adults with BED, 63% reported a weight problem (average onset age, 12.2 years) before engaging in binge eating and dieting.[57] Of the participants who began dieting, 21% became overweight and then progressed to binge eating, whereas 16% started binge eating, became overweight, and then began dieting. Additional risk factors for BED include the development of unhealthy eating patterns (eg, eating too much, too little, or choosing high-caloric foods over healthy alternatives) and poor weight control habits (eg, extreme dieting, caloric restriction, purging, or smoking).[58,59]

Family, Social, and Cultural Factors

Adults, primarily females, with less than a high school education, who live in poverty and who have been raised in a large family with limited parental support are at greater risk for obesity.[60] Within a larger social setting, obese adults face stigmatization and discrimination, and these experiences affect mental health. More frequent exposure to stigmatization correlates with greater psychological distress, more avoidance behaviors, and higher levels of self-criticism. These factors—distress, avoidance, and self-criticism—are associated with greater obesity.[30]

MENTAL HEALTH ASSESSMENT OF OBESE CHILDREN, ADOLESCENTS, AND ADULTS

Body-Image Assessments and Self-Esteem

Obese children and adults who have body-image dissatisfaction are at greater risk for mental health disorders and severe obesity, so screening tools for body image and self-worth are useful in identifying this risk. Conversely, moderate levels of body-image dissatisfaction can be a motivating factor in weight loss for some. A number of questionnaires are available to determine the level of comfort or discomfort with body shape and size for adults and adolescents (**Table 2**). The Body-Image Questionnaires, used with overweight adolescents and adults, assess the level of body-image dissatisfaction and self-perceived ideal weight.[61] The Rosenberg Self-esteem Scale, a brief 10-item questionnaire, measures self-worth and self-acceptance.

Emotions, Moods, and Psychosocial Functioning

A second area for assessment is emotions and moods, eating disorders, and other psychosocial functioning. Screening tools for depression, anxiety, and ADHD, especially with children, identify areas of mental health risks for overweight children and adults. Since depression has limited association with overweight children and adults, it may be most helpful in assessing patients with the greatest psychological barriers, which impede weight loss treatments. The Beck's Depression Inventory II and the

Table 2
Mental health screening tools for overweight and obese individuals

Assessment Tools	Age Range	Description
Eating Disorder Examination Questionnaire/Youth Eating Disorder Examination Questionnaire	EDE-Q sixth-grade reading level or higher YEDE-Q Children under sixth-grade reading level	EDE-Q 36-item self-report measure that assesses eating disorder psychopathology, restraint, eating concerns, weight control concerns, and shape concerns
Body-Image Assessment for Obesity	Adults	18 silhouettes of male and female who range from very thin to obese Assesses for discrepancy between current, ideal, and reasonable body size
Rosenberg Self-Esteem Scale	Adolescents and adults	10-item self-report that measures self-worth and self-acceptance
SF-36 Health Survey	14–Adult	36-item measure that assesses quality of life as related to physical and mental health
Dutch Eating Behavior Questionnaire—Restraint Scale	9–Adult	Restraint Scale assesses 3 eating behaviors: restrained eating, emotional eating, and external eating
Children's Eating Behavior Inventory	Children 2–12 y of age	40-questionnaire parent report measure to assess mealtime problems in children related to food preference/dislikes, compliance during meals, self-feeding skills, and family member's perception of stress during mealtime
Questionnaire on Eating and Weight Patterns—Revised	Adolescents and adults	28-item questionnaire to assess for BED
Beck Depression Inventory Patient Health Questionnaire-9	fifth- or sixth-grade reading level Adults	21-item assessment for depression symptoms 9-item depression screening tool for primary care patients

Abbreviations: EDE-Q, Eating Disorder Examination Questionnaire; YEDE-Q, Youth Eating Disorder Examination Questionnaire.

9-item depression scale of the Patient Health Questionnaire are standardized assessments for depression. Quality-of life measures such as the short form 36-item (SF-36) questionnaire assess physical and mental health functioning.

Another useful tool, a food monitoring system, gathers information on the psychosocial aspects of eating. Food monitoring charts are designed to track the behavioral aspects of eating patterns in relationship to environmental triggers, emotional states, and thoughts. Parental involvement is crucial for accomplishing this type of behavioral monitoring for children and adolescents. Food diaries typically log time of day, type and quantity of food consumed, social triggers, emotions, self-control, and thoughts. Moreover, food diaries may not be accurate in children younger than 10 years due to lack of skills.[6] With children, the Behavior Eating Test (BET) and Bob and Tom's Method of Assessing Nutrition (BATMAN) assess food-related thoughts and behaviors.[6] BET monitors the choice of high- and low-calorie foods and observes the quantity of food eaten. BATMAN identifies psychosocial factors that affect eating. The child's eating behaviors and the parents' response to the behavior are recorded. With this information, individual treatment plans and recommendations for the parents, which include behavioral interventions, meal plans, attitude changes toward food, and modifying reactions to eating behaviors, are developed.

For adults, assessing eating patterns sets the foundation for developing a weight loss plan. Food intake is assessed in 3 areas: number of times the individual eats per day, calories, and types of food consumed. Obese individuals may underestimate food consumption by as much as 50%,[62] In addition to tracking the number of times an individual eats per day, the log should include the frequency, timing, and feelings of the person when eating. This assessment provides patterns of eating that interfere with efforts to lose weight or just halt weight gain. The pattern may reveal that eating is tied to specific emotions, such as boredom, anxiety, tiredness, stress, anger, depression, happiness, or loneliness. The next step includes targeting emotions for a behavioral or interpersonal therapeutic intervention along with designing a structured meal plan.[50]

Binge Eating Disorder Assessment

Assessing for BED is of particular concern because of its close correlation with obesity and weight loss difficulties. Questionnaires and clinical interviewing strategies help clarify binge eating behaviors that affect the individual's obesity (see **Table 2**). After collecting general information, including family history of obesity, mental illness, and onset of overweight/obesity, a behavioral assessment of eating behaviors helps identify binge eating patterns, such as consuming large quantities of foods in short periods of time and feeling out of control with eating. If binge eating is diagnosed, screening for body-image concerns, mood/anxiety disorders, quality of life, self-efficacy, and current stressful events should be considered, because these factors can be barriers that interfere with treatment.[50]

MENTAL HEALTH TREATMENT AND OBESE ADULTS

Since obesity treatment is a key component in health care, it is important to understand how mental health and obesity treatment, along with weight loss through dieting or surgery, are related. Mental health factors, emotions, behaviors, and social contexts that enhance or hinder weight loss must be taken into consideration. Adults who are able to maintain weight loss tend to be internalizers and optimistic.[55] Adults who are able to set realistic goals, have a sense of confidence, have an internal drive to monitor their eating, and exhibit a healthy sense of body image and self-worth are able to maintain weight loss. Adults who regain weight tend to be externalizers and pessimistic; they blame medical conditions for their weight, focus on obstacles to weight loss, feel more subjective hunger, and set rigid eating rules but lose control in their eating and tend to be emotional and stress eaters. The factors that are primarily associated with the psychological characteristics of patients who maintain their weight loss and those who regain weight are listed in **Box 2**.[55] Adults who are reward dependent, warm, dedicated, attached, cooperative, tolerant, helpful, and compassionate are more likely to participate in a weight loss program. In addition, adults who are successful at weight loss have lower novelty seeking behaviors, which means that they are less impulsive, extravagant, and have fewer disorderly characteristics than those of adults with unsuccessful weight loss.

In a review of weight loss treatment clinical trials with at least 1-year follow-up, weight loss programs with intensive counseling and behavior therapy interventions demonstrate the most success for patients; however, weight loss is modest.[63] In these programs, a majority of the interventions consist of frequent contact with a health care provider or allied health specialist (eg, monthly for 3–6 months) and include behavioral techniques, such as self-monitoring, activity schedules, stress management, and social support.

For the majority of those who undergo bariatric surgery, a positive impact exists on quality of life—both physical and mental health functioning, which includes less depression, improved self-esteem, and positive psychosocial functioning.[64] However, a significant number of obesity surgery patients (20%–30%) regain weight after 2 years.[65] Since many severely obese patients have diagnoses according to the Diagnostic and Statistical Manual of Mental Disorders (between 22% and 47%), results indicate that patients with severe psychiatric conditions (eg, prior psychiatric hospitalization, suicidal ideation, and major psychosocial stressors) have the poorest outcomes.[64] "Distress based on serious psychiatric disturbance is probably an impediment to obesity surgery, whereas distress based on the experience of being

Box 2
Psychological characteristics of weight maintenance and weight regain

Weight Maintenance	Weight Regain
Achievable weight loss goal	Attribution of obesity to medical factors
Flexible control over eating	Perceiving barriers to weight loss behaviors
Self-monitoring	Novelty seeking
Self-efficacy	Weight cycling
Autonomy	Disinhibited eating
"Health narcissism"	More hunger
Motivated and confident in losing weight	Binge eating
Stability in life	Eating in response to negative emotions and stress
Capacity for close relationships	Psychosocial stressors
	Lack of social support
	Passive reaction to problems
	Lack of confidence
	Black/white thinking

morbidly obese is probably a positive predictor of outcome.[64]" Binge eating and eating to reduce stress, boredom, or coping with emotions also have a negative impact on weight loss.[55]

Overall, obese adults do not suffer from depression, anxiety, or other mental health issues any more than normal weight adults unless they are in the extreme ranges of obesity. Lower body-image satisfaction, stigmatizing experiences, lower SES, and poor self-esteem are correlated with more severe ranges of obesity in adults. Obese adults who successfully lose weight either through weight loss programs or surgery report a significant improvement in mental health and psychosocial functioning. The majority of these research studies are based on women, and few studies have focused specifically on the unique characteristics of men, obesity, and mental health.

Mental Health Treatment of Body Image and Self-Esteem in Obese Individuals

Body-image dissatisfaction in overweight and obese individuals has a negative impact on psychosocial functioning. Cognitive-behavioral therapy (CBT) is one mental health treatment model that helps to improve body-image dissatisfaction by focusing on the cognitions, emotions, and behaviors that contribute to body-image dissatisfaction.[66] CBT improves not just body-image satisfaction but also self-esteem and overeating. The goal is to change the thought process toward a more positive way of evaluating the individual's self-worth and his or her relationship to food.[67] This, in turn, expands the cognitive and behavioral choices the individual has regarding self-esteem and body image. CBT treatments include self-monitoring techniques, challenging automatic thoughts and beliefs, correcting distorted thoughts, body-image desensitization, and relaxation techniques. Additionally, *The Body Image Workbook: An Eight-Step Program for Learning to Like Your Looks* is a useful self-help resource that may serve as an adjunctive intervention to CBT therapy.[68]

Similarly, mindfulness meditation improves body-image dissatisfaction by replacing negative images and thinking with self-acceptance, a nonjudging attitude, and openness toward the range of emotions and possibilities that arise throughout the day. Focused breathing and relaxation techniques are employed to lessen anxiety and to physiologically relax the body. The mindfulness aids in recreating body-image experiences, transforming perceptions, and developing compassion for one's self, while providing an opportunity to remove previously established schemas, core beliefs, automatic thoughts, and behaviors that maintain body-image dissatisfaction.[69]

Another mental health treatment approach focuses on self-esteem improvement and not on diet at all. In the diet group, 51% of the adults felt better about themselves, whereas 93% of the nondiet group reported higher self-esteem.[70] The nondieting approaches do not produce the same weight loss results as low-calorie diets and physical activity but are effective for long-term changes in self-esteem and self-worth.[70] Nondieting approaches aim to enhance body acceptance, self-esteem, and physical activity; integrate off limit foods; decrease calorie restriction; and provide education on the adverse effects of diets, weight cycling, and biologic influences on obesity.[70] Moreover, nondieting approaches teach individuals to identify hunger and fullness cues to help guide eating.[71]

Mood Disorder Treatment and Obesity

Overweight and obese individuals who have depression, anxiety, or bipolar disorder should receive treatment for these conditions. Left untreated, these psychological disorders can interfere with weight loss success and put the individual at risk for treatment drop out.[72] Mood disorders are successfully treated with CBT in individual and group therapy or with self-help materials. The *Feeling Good Handbook* and *Mind Over*

Mood are CBT-based interventions and self-directed workbooks that are useful in the treatment of mood disorders.[73,74]

Treating Emotional Eating in Overweight and Obese Individuals

Overweight and obese individuals may be triggered to engage in unhealthy eating behaviors by stress, emotions, or trauma. Often, adults use overeating to mask and distract themselves from intense and uncomfortable emotional experiences. Eating allows the individual to avoid negative feelings and cope with the intensity of the emotions. Mental health treatments such as CBT address the connections between food and feelings and provide new ways to cope with emotions, stress, or trauma.[75] On the other hand, if CBT is unsuccessful, Dialectical-Behavioral Therapy (DBT) can be tried as an alternative approach. However, DBT should not be a first line of treatment, because it is an intensive, long-term treatment.[75] DBT, traditionally a treatment of borderline personality, has recently been used for disordered eating in individualized or skills training groups. Individual DBT therapy targets the following areas: decreasing high-risk suicidal behavior, decreasing treatment-interfering behaviors such as BED, decreasing behaviors that interfere with quality of life and post-traumatic stress responses, increasing self-respect, and obtaining new coping and interpersonal skills.[76] The skills training group focuses on learning coping and interpersonal skills necessary to ameliorate behaviors contributing to disordered eating and emotional regulation. There are 4 modules that concentrate on mindfulness, interpersonal effectiveness, distress tolerance, and emotional regulation.[76]

Mental Health Treatment for Overweight and Obese with Binge Eating Disorder

The most effective treatments for BED in overweight or obese individuals are CBT and Interpersonal therapy (IPT). These interventions aim to change behaviors, emotions, and interpersonal skills affecting weight gain, BED, and weight loss maintenance. CBT and IPT reduce binges and other comorbid disorders. On the other hand, CBT and IPT do not produce significant weight loss but rather tackle the issues that make weight loss difficult for some individuals.[77] CBT provides education on obesity and nutrition; helps to modify eating and food choices; and tracks eating, emotions, mood, self-esteem, and body dissatisfaction as related to episodes of binge eating.[67]

IPT is validated as an effective treatment for BED.[78] IPT is a short-term therapy that focuses on the role of interpersonal functioning in the evolution and maintenance of the BED. It does not focus directly on the symptoms but rather the interplay between the environment (ie, parents/peers), body image, self-esteem, and disordered eating.[79] IPT pinpoints 4 areas—grief, role transition, role disputes, and interpersonal deficits—that are explored and changed through improving mood, self-esteem, feelings of empowerment, and ability to change. The changes made in treatment are designed to decrease the frequency of binges and improve self-esteem.[79]

Finally, mindfulness meditation as an intervention has shown success in treating BED. A 6-week trial showed that mindful meditation helps to reduce the number of binges, improves sense of control, and improves ability to recognize hunger and fullness cues, depression, and anxiety.[80] Mindfulness meditation is a technique that allows the individual to bring focus to the environment with a detached sense of awareness. The individual is taught to strive for a nonjudging and self-accepting attitude. Consequently, this provides a sense of relaxation and teaches the individual to tolerate distressing emotions that may lead to binge eating.[81] The focus of awareness can also be used to recognize cues for hunger and fullness, which combat overeating and bingeing.

Treatment Considerations for Weight Loss Surgery with the Severely Obese

In the severely obese, weight loss surgery may be the most effective treatment for weight loss to improve the individual's health. In a 4-year follow-up study of individuals who had surgical weight loss, psychosocial functioning dramatically improved.[82] Severely obese individuals, to benefit from the weight loss surgery, need to be able to comply with the demands of postsurgery diet and behavioral changes.[71] The mental health factors that affect weight loss in overweight and obese individuals can also complicate a severely obese individual's aptitude to succeed postsurgery. In postsurgery individuals, pre-existing BED is related to weight gain and worse mental health.[83] Furthermore, emotional eating can lead to binge eating and undermine the weight loss effort.

For postsurgery success, an individual should complete a psychological evaluation. The evaluation can determine the existence of mental health issues, coping skills, personality traits, self-esteem, body dissatisfaction, interpersonal skills, along with levels of motivation, and readiness for change that would interfere with postsurgery weight loss. The presence of these factors needs to be addressed before and after the surgery to create the elements vital for weight loss and maintenance. Furthermore, addressing these mental health factors allows for psychological and behavioral changes that will promote long-term lifestyle changes.[55]

MENTAL HEALTH AND OBESITY PREVENTION

Preventive measures are needed to decrease the obesity epidemic in the United States. Although prevention protocols with children have not yet made an impact on obesity rates, early intervention with children and adolescents who are already overweight or obese has shown to decrease the likelihood of adult obesity.[84] Screening for additional factors, such as body-image dissatisfaction, unhealthy weight control habits, depression, low self-esteem, stigmatizing experiences, environment, and BED, in overweight children and adolescents can help identify the focus of treatment and have an impact on weight loss and maintenance. Unhealthy weight control and body-image dissatisfaction are highly common in adolescents and should be regularly screened. Intervening early may allow children and adolescents to change behaviors before patterns become more ingrained and, thus, more difficult to change as adults.[22] In addition, family and community-focused interventions are being implemented in many settings. There are new initiatives where health providers are linking with other community resources—recreation centers, schools, and food centers. Advocacy for nutritional options in schools and communities, especially low-income communities, is receiving more attention. Change is needed in enhancing physical activity for children, adolescents, adults, and seniors. We are still in the infancy stage of addressing the obesity epidemic, and new ideas are spawning throughout the country. National Initiative for Children's Healthcare Quality (www.nichq.org/nichq) has a host of models of obesity programs that are being offered. These interventions build on the systemic aspects of prevention and attend to the social-emotional and cultural aspects of obesity.

SUMMARY

Obesity is a stronger predictor of poor physical health but not poor mental health. Overall, obese individuals do not suffer from depression, anxiety, or other mental health issues any more than normal weight individuals unless they are in the extreme ranges of obesity. Lower body-image satisfaction, mood disorders, binge eating or other disordered eating behaviors, and poor self-esteem must be addressed with referrals to appropriate mental health specialists. Treatment options that may improve these underlying comorbid disorders are available, which, in the long run, may improve psychological functioning and weight loss.

REFERENCES

1. US Department of Health and Human Services, Centers for Disease Control and Prevention. Overweight and obesity trends among adults. Available at: http://www.cdc.gov/nccdphp/dnpa/obesity/trend/index.htm. Accessed June 1, 2008.
2. Wardle J, Cooke L. The impact of obesity on psychological well-being. Best Pract Res Clin Endocrinol Metab 2005;19:421–40.
3. Padgett J, Biro FM. Different shapes in different culture: body dissatisfaction, overweight, and obesity in African-American and Caucasian females. J Pediatr Adolesc Gynecol 2003;16(6):349–54.
4. Vander Wal JS. Eating and body image concerns among average weight and obese African American and Hispanic girls. Eat Behav 2004;5(2):181–7.
5. Jansen W, vandeLooij-Jansen PM, de Wilde EF, et al. Feeling fat rather than being fat may be associated with psychological well-being in young Dutch adolescents. J Adolesc Health 2007;42:128–36.
6. Netemeyer S, Williamson D. Assessment of eating disturbance in children and adolescents with eating disorders and obesity. In: Thompson J, Smolak L, editors. Bodyimage, eating disorders, and obesity in youth. Washington, DC: APA; 2001. p. 215–33.
7. French SA, Story M, Perry CL. Self-esteem and obesity in children and adolescents: a literature review. Obes Res 1995;3:479–90.
8. Young-Hyman D, Schlundt DG, Herman-Wenderoth L, et al. Obesity, appearance, and psychosocial adaptation in young African American children. J Pediatr Psychol 2003;28(7):463–72.
9. Melnyk BM, Small L, Morrison-Beedy D, et al. Mental health correlates of healthy lifestyle attitudes, beliefs, choices, and behaviors in overweight adolescents. J Pediatr Health Care 2006;3(4):401–6.
10. Levine M, Smolak L. Media as context for the development of disordered eating. In: Levine M, Smolak L, Striegel-Moore R, editors. Developmental psychopathology of eating disorders. Hillsdale (NJ): Erlbaum; 1996. p. 235–57.
11. Must A, Strauss RS. Risk and consequences of childhood and adolescent obesity. Int J Obes 1999;2(Suppl 2):S2–11.
12. Anderson SE, Cohenp P, Naumova EN, et al. Association of depression and anxiety disorders with weight change in a prospective community based study of children followed up into adulthood. Arch Pediatr Adolesc Med 2006;160: 285–91.
13. Swallen KC, Reither EN, Haas SA, et al. Overweight, obesity and health related quality of life among adolescents: the national longitudinal study of adolescent health. Pediatrics 2005;115:340–7.
14. Zametkin AJ, Zoon CK, Klein HW, et al. Psychiatric aspects of children and adolescent obesity: a review of the past 10 years. J Am Acad Child Adolesc Psychiatry 2004;43(2):134–50.
15. Goodman E, Whitaker RC. A prospective study of the role of depression in the development and persistence of adolescent obesity. Pediatrics 2002;110: 497–504.

16. Cortese S, Isnard P, Frelut ML, et al. Association between symptoms of attention-deficit hyperactivity disorder and bulimic behaviors in a clinical sample of severely obese adolescents. Int J Obes 2007;31:340–6.
17. Center for Disease Control (CDC). Available at: www.cdc.gov/nccdphp/dnpa/obesity/trend/maps; 2008. Accessed October 20, 2008.
18. Drewnowski A, Specter SE. Poverty and obesity: the role of energy density and energy costs. Am J Clin Nutr 2004;79:6–16.
19. Miech RA, Kumanyika SK, Stettler N, et al. Trends in the association of poverty with overweight among US Adolescents. JAMA 2006;295(20):2385–93.
20. Sothern MS, Gordon ST. Prevention of obesity in young children: a critical challenge for medical professionals. Clin Pediatr 2003;42:101–11.
21. Mamun AA, Lawlor DA, O'Callaghan JF, et al. Family and early life factors associated with changes in overweight status between ages 5 and 14 years: findings from the Mater University Study of pregnancy and its outcomes. Int J Obes 2005;29:475–82.
22. AAP. Policy statement: prevention of pediatric overweight and obesity. Pediatrics 2003;112(2):424–30.
23. Birch LL, Davison KK. Family environmental factors influencing the developing behavioral controls of food intake and childhood overweight. Pediatr Clin North Am 2001;48(4):893–907.
24. Lindsey AC, Sussner KM, Kim J, et al. The role of parents in preventing childhood obesity. Future Child 2006;16(1):169–86.
25. Dennison BA, Erb TA, Jenkins PI. Television viewing and television in bedroom associated with overweight risk among low-income preschool children. Pediatrics 2002;109(6):1028–35.
26. Wiecha JL, Sobol AM, Peterson KE, et al. Household television access: associations with screen time, reading and homework among youth. Ambul Pediatr 2001;1(5):244–51.
27. Gillman MW, Rifas-Shiman SL, Frazier AL, et al. Family dinner and diet quality among older children, adolescents and adults. Arch Fam Med 2000;9(3):235–40.
28. Fogelholm M, Nuutinen O, Pasanen M, et al. Parent-child relationship of physical activity patterns and obesity. Int J Obes 1999;23(12):1262–78.
29. Puhl RM, Latner JD. Stigma, obesity, and the health of the Nation's children. Psychol Bull 2007;133(4):557–80.
30. Myers A, Rosen JC. Obesity, stigmatization and coping: relation to mental health symptoms, body image, and self-esteem. Int J Obes 1999;23:221–30.
31. Wilfley DE, Tibbs TL, VanBuren DJ, et al. Lifestyle intervention in the treatment of childhood overweight: a meta-analytic review of randomized controlled trials. Health Psychol 2007;26(5):521–32.
32. Epstein LH, Paluch RA, Roennich JN, et al. Family-based obesity treatment, then and now: twenty-five years of pediatric obesity treatment. Health Psychol 2007;26(4):381–91.
33. Golan M, Crow S. Parents are key players in the prevention and treatment of weight-related problems. Nutr Rev 2004;62(1):39–50.
34. Jelalian E, Saelen BE. Empirically supported treatments in pediatric psychology: pediatric obesity. J Pediatr Psychol 1999;24(3):223–48.
35. Kamath CC, Vickers KS, Ehrlich A, et al. Behavioral interventions to prevent childhood obesity. A systematic review and meta-analyses of randomized trials. J Clin Endocrinol Metab 2008;10:2006–411.
36. American Academy of Pediatrics. Available at: www.aap.org. Accessed October 20, 2008.

37. Wertheim EH, Paxton SJ, Blaney S. Risk factors for the development of body image disturbances. In: Thompson JK, editor. Handbook of eating disorders and obesity. Hoboken (NJ): John Wiley & Sons, Inc; 2004. p. 463–514.
38. Mond JM, Rodgers B, Hay P, et al. Obesity and impairment in psychosocial functioning in women: the mediating role of eating disorders. Obesity 2007;15: 2769–79.
39. Friedman KE, Reichmann SK, Costanzo PR, et al. Body image partially mediates the relationship between obesity and psychological distress. Obes Res 2002; 10(33):41.
40. McCabe M, Ricciardelli M. Weight and shape concerns of boys and men. In: Thompson JK, editor. Handbook of eating disorders and obesity. Hoboken (NJ): John Wiley & Sons, Inc; 2004. p. 606–34.
41. Onyike CU, Crum RM, Lee HB, et al. Is obesity associated with major depression? Results from the Third National health and nutrition examination survey. Am J Epidemiol 2003;158:1139–47.
42. Dixon JB, Dixon MC, O'Brien PE. Depression in association with severe obesity. Arch Intern Med 2003;163(20):58–65.
43. Jia H, Lubetkin EI. The impact of obesity on health-related quality of life in the general adult US population. J Publ Health 2005;27(2):156–64. Available at: www.reuters.com/article. Accessed June 2008.
44. Callegari A, Michelini I, Sguazzin C, et al. Efficacy of the SF-36 questionnaire, in identifying obese patients with psychological discomfort. Obes Surg 2005;15: 254–60.
45. Doll HA, Petersen SEK, Stewart-Brown SL. Obesity and physical and emotional well-being: associations between BMI, chronic illness, and the physical and mental components of the SF-36 questionnaire. Obes Res 2000;8(2):160–70.
46. Huang I-C, Fangakis C, Wu AW. The relationship of excess body weight and health-related quality of life: evidence from a population study in Taiwan. Int J Obes 2006;30:1250–9.
47. Han TS, Tijhuis MAR, Lean MEJ, et al. Quality of life in relation to overweight and body fat distribution. Am J Public Health 1998;88(12):1814–20.
48. Dickerson FB, Brown CH, Kreyenbuhl JA, et al. Obesity among individuals with serious mental illness. Acta Psychiatr Scand 2006;113:306–13.
49. Sullian S, Cloninger CR, Przybeck TR, et al. Personality characteristics in obesity and relationship with successful weight loss. Int J Obes 2007;31:669–74.
50. Phelan S, Wadden TA. Behavioral assessment of obesity. In: Thompson JK, editor. Handbook of eating disorders and obesity. Hoboken (NJ): John Wiley & Sons, Inc; 2004. p. 393–420.
51. Raymond NC, Bartholome LT, Lee SS, et al. A comparison of energy intake and food selection during laboratory binge eating episodes in obese women with and without binge eating disorder diagnosis. Int J Eat Disord 2007;40:67–71.
52. Walsh B, Wilfley DE, Stein RI, et al. Binge eating disorder. Brochure prepared for continuing education through the University of South Florida and the Academy for Eating Disorders 2003.
53. Rieger E, Wilfley DE, Stein RI, et al. A comparison of quality of life in obese individuals with and without binge eating disorder. Int J Eat Disord 2005;37:234–40.
54. Wadden T, Foster GD, Brownell KD, et al. Obesity: responding to the global epidemic. J Consult Clin Psychol 2002;70:510–29.
55. Elfhag K, Rossner S. Who succeeds in maintaining weight loss? A conceptual review of factors associated with weight loss maintenance and weight regain. Obes Rev 2005;6(67):85.

56. Strober M. Disorders of the self in anorexia nervosa. In: Johnson C, editor. Psychodynamic treatment of anorexia nervosa and bulimia. New York: Guilford; 1991. p. 354–73.
57. Reas DL, Grilo CM. Timing and sequence of the onset of overweight, dieting, and binge eating in overweight patients with binge eating disorder. Int J Eat Disord 2007;40:165–70.
58. Marcus MD, Moulton MM, Greeno CG. Binge eating disorder onset in obese patients with binge eating disorder. Addict Behav 1995;20:747–55.
59. Decaluwe V, Braet C, Fairburn CG. Binge eating in obese children and adolescents. Int J Eat Disord 2003;22:78–84.
60. Rohrer JE, Rohland BM. Psychosocial risk factors for obesity among women in a family planning clinic. BMC Fam Pract 2004;5:20.
61. Stewart TM, Williamson DA. Assessment of body image disturbance. In: Thompson JK, editor. Handbook of eating disorders and obesity. Hoboken (NJ): John Wiley & Sons, Inc; 2004. p. 495–514.
62. Lichtman SW, Pisarska K, Berman ER, et al. Discrepancy between self-reported and actual caloric intake and exercise in obese subjects. N Engl J Med 1992; 327(27):1893–8 As cited in: Phelan S, Wadden TA. Behavioral assessment of obesity. In: Thompson JK, editor. Handbook of eating disorders and obesity. Hoboken (NJ): John Wiley & Sons, Inc; 2004;393–420.
63. McTigue KM, Harris R, Hemphill B, et al. Screening and interventions for obesity in adults: summary of the evidence for the US preventive services task force. Ann Intern Med 2003;139(11):933–50.
64. Herpertz S, Kielmann R, Wolf AM, et al. Do psychosocial variables predict weight loss or mental health after obesity surgery? A systematic review. Obes Res 2004; 12(10):1154–569.
65. Hsu LKG. Nonsurgical factors that influence the outcome of bariatric surgery: a review. Psychosom Med 1998;60(3):338–46.
66. Cash TF, Hrabosky JI. Treatment of body image disturbances. In: Thompson JK, editor. Handbook of eating disorders and obesity. Hoboken (NJ): John Wiley & Sons, Inc; 2004. p. 515–41.
67. Fairburn C, Marcus MD, Wilson GT, et al. Cognitive behavioral therapy for binge eating and bulimia nervosa. In: Fairburn C, Wilson GT, editors. Binge eating. New York: Guilford Press; 1993. p. 361–404.
68. Cash TF. The body image workbook: an eight-step program for learning to like your looks. Oakland (CA): New Harbinger; 2008. p. 1–216.
69. Stewart T. Light on body image treatment: acceptance through mindfulness. Behav Modif 2004;28:783–811.
70. Bacon L, Keim NL, Van Loan MD, et al. Evaluating a 'non-diet' wellness intervention for improvement of metabolic fitness, psychological well-being and eating and activity behaviors. Int J Obes 2002;26:854–65.
71. Sarwer DB, Foster GD, Wadden TA. Treatment of obesity I: adult obesity. In: Thompson JK, editor. Handbook of eating disorders and obesity. Hoboken (NJ): John Wiley & Sons, Inc; 2004. p. 421–42.
72. Clark MM, Niaura R, King TK, et al. Depression, smoking, activity level, and health status: pretreatment predictors of attrition in obesity treatment. Addict Behav 1996;21(4):509–13.
73. Burns DD. The feeling good handbook. New York: Plume; 1999. p. 1–768.
74. Greenberger D, Padesky C. Mind over mood: change how you feel by changing the way you think. New York: Guilford Press; 1995. p. 1–243.

75. Blocher McCabe E, LaVia MC, Marcus MD. Dialectical behavioral therapy for eating disorders. In: Thompson JK, editor. Handbook of eating disorders and obesity. Hoboken (NJ): John Wiley & Sons, Inc; 2004. p. 232–44.
76. Linehan M. Cognitive-behavioral treatment of borderline personality disorder. New York: NY; The Guilford Press; 1993. p. 1–558.
77. Munsch S, Biedert E, Meyer A, et al. A randomized comparison of cognitive behavioral therapy and behavioral weight loss treatment for overweight individuals with binge eating disorder. Int J Eat Disord 2007;40(2):102–13.
78. Peterson CB, Mitchell JE. Psychosocial and pharmacological treatment of eating disorders: a review of research findings. J Clin Psychol 1999;55(6):685–97.
79. Tantleff-Dunn S, Goke-LaRose J, Peterson RD. Interpersonal psychotherapy for the treatment of anorexia nervosa, bulimia nervosa, and binge eating disorder. In: Thompson JK, editor. Handbook of eating disorders and obesity. Hoboken (NJ): John Wiley & Sons, Inc; 2004. p. 163–85.
80. Kristeller J, Hallett C. An exploratory study of a meditation-based intervention for binge eating disorder. J Health Psychol 1999;4:356–63.
81. Kabat-Zinn J. Full catastrophe living: using the wisdom of your body and mind to face stress, pain, and illness. 15th edition. New York: Delta Trade Paperback/Bantam Dell; 2005.
82. Karlsson J, Taft C, Sjostrom L, et al. Psychosocial functioning in the obese before and after weight reduction: construct validity and responsiveness of the obesity-related problems scale. Int J Obes 2003;27:617–30.
83. Larsen JK, Greenen R, Ramshorst BV, et al. Binge eating and exercise behavior after surgery for severe obesity: a structural equation model. Int J Eat Disord 2006;39:369–75.
84. Cooperberg J, Faith M. Treatment of obesity II: childhood and adolescent obesity. In: Thompson JK, editor. Handbook of eating disorders and obesity. Hoboken (NJ): John Wiley & Sons, Inc; 2004. p. 443–60.

The Obesity Epidemic: Are Minority Individuals Equally Affected?

Pablo J. Calzada, DO, MPH, FAAFP*, Paula Anderson-Worts, DO, MPH

KEYWORDS

- Obesity • Minorities • Etiology
- Genetic makeup • Psychosocial • Socioeconomic
- Access and quality of health care • Intervention strategies

EPIDEMIOLOGY

Despite its prevalence in all segments of the American population, obesity imposes a larger burden on, and poses a larger threat to, minority populations. Statistics show that overweight and obesity occur disproportionately among minorities and those of lower socioeconomic status. Epidemiologic data demonstrate that ethnic and racial minorities have a greater prevalence of obesity compared with that in whites (**Fig. 1**).[1] It has been estimated that by the year 2040, minority groups will make up more than 50% of the overall US population. This fact may be a predictor of the potential devastation obesity will pose to the health status of all Americans if ignored.

Minority and low-socioeconomic-status groups are disproportionately affected at all ages. Annual increases in prevalence of obesity ranged from 0.3 to 0.9 percentage points across groups. It is estimated that by 2015, 75% of adults will be overweight or obese, and 41% will be obese. Weight gain is particularly detrimental to Asians. Data suggest that the inverse association of a healthy diet with diabetes is stronger for minorities than that for Caucasians. The risk of diabetes is significantly higher among Asians, Hispanics, and African Americans than that among Caucasians before and after taking into account differences in body mass index (BMI).

One-third of women in the United States are affected by the obesity epidemic. Minority women are at highest risk, with females of African American or Hispanic ethnicity having close to 50% obesity rate. Obesity significantly increases risk for mortality and morbidity in women. Of further concern, there is strong evidence that maternal adiposity increases the risk of obesity in the offspring through perinatal mechanisms, perpetuating this disease process.[2]

Department of Family Medicine and Public Health, Nova Southeastern University College of Osteopathic Medicine, 3200 S. University Drive, Davie, FL 33328-2018, USA
* Corresponding author.
E-mail address: calzada@nsu.nova.edu (P.J. Calzada).

Prim Care Clin Office Pract 36 (2009) 307–317
doi:10.1016/j.pop.2009.01.007 **primarycare.theclinics.com**

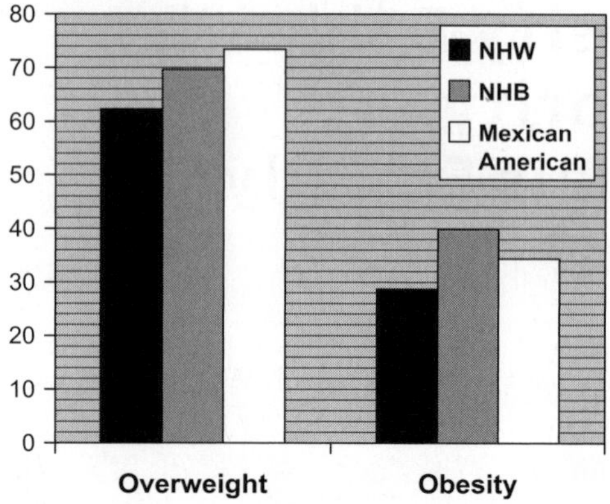

Fig. 1. Prevalence of obesity by race and ethnicity. NHB, non-Hispanic black; NHW, non-Hispanic white.

OBESITY IN OLDER MINORITIES AND CHILDREN

The effects of obesity do not discriminate; they have affected the health of both young and old. Elderly members of minority groups, a rapidly growing population in the United States, are adversely affected by the increased prevalence of obesity and all comorbid factors directly and indirectly associated with excessive weight.[3] Excessive weight negatively affects the progression of many degenerative diseases seen in older adults. As excessive weight increases, morbidity and mortality of chronic diseases escalate in the elderly population. Available treatments include lifestyle modification programs, with a focus on eating a healthy diet and increasing physical activity, and possibly adjunctive pharmacotherapy.[2] Because reducing morbidity through health promotion and disease prevention could both improve the quality of elderly life and lessen the burden on the health care system, it would seem reasonable that such efforts, including nutrition education, in minority elderly would be of great benefit. The extent of the potential value of such preventive programs, however, remains uncertain. The task of determining the nutrient needs of the elderly is difficult. Special studies are required to describe the association of nutrition-related factors with chronic diseases, particularly those prevalent in minority elders.[3]

Rising trends in overweight and obesity in children are confirmed in developed as well as in developing countries. Available estimates for the period between the 1980s and 1990s show the prevalence of overweight and obesity in children increased by a magnitude of 2 to 5 times in developed countries (e.g., from 11% to more than 30% in boys in Canada), and up to almost 4 times in developing countries (e.g., from 4% to 14% in Brazil).[4] Additionally, data indicate that children from ethnic minorities in Europe are more frequently overweight or obese than European children. For Europeans, social class status and the average family length of stay after immigration have also proven to be factors that may influence the pattern of overweight and obesity in children at school entry.[5]

In the past 10 years, there has been a tremendous increase in the number of studies examining the etiology and health effects of obesity in children.[6] Overweight children aged between 6 and 11 years have more than doubled, whereas the incidence for adolescents from age 12 to 19 years has tripled between 1980 and 2000. It is clear that children and adolescents from ethnic minorities and rural low-income populations bear an excess burden of obesity and its related comorbidities, as childhood obesity is more prevalent among minority subgroups, such as African Americans and Hispanics

(**Fig. 2**).[7] In fact, there is strong evidence that overweight has increased fastest among minorities, creating large demographic differences in the prevalence of children who are overweight. As in the adult population, childhood and adolescent overweight and obesity are related to the development of acute and chronic medical conditions, increased health risks and, ultimately, increased risk of adult obesity, with its negative implications on morbidity and mortality rates. Although these health concerns are relevant to all children, they affect minority groups to a greater extent.

Overweight increased significantly and steadily among African American, Hispanic, and white children between 1986 and 1998. By the year 1998, overweight prevalence increased to 21.5% among African Americans, 21.8% among Hispanics, and 12.3% among non-Hispanic whites. In addition, overweight children were heavier in 1998 compared with 1986. The number of children with BMI greater than the 85th percentile increased significantly from 1986 to 1998 among African American and Hispanic children and not significantly among white children.[8]

The increased representation of overweight or obese youth among minority groups and low-income populations seems to mimic the excess morbidity of overweight- and obesity-induced health conditions in adults of the same population group. Reasons for the racial and ethnic disparity in childhood obesity are unclear. Many factors are probably involved, including environmental and genetic factors. Differences in lifestyle behaviors and family characteristics might help to explain some of these subgroup differences starting at an early age. Low-income and minority children watch more television than white, nonpoor children and are potentially exposed to more commercials advertising high-calorie, low-nutrient food during an average hour of television programming.[9] Studies suggest that Hispanic and African American children have lower aerobic fitness levels than those of Caucasian children, and this effect is independent of gender, maturation, and body composition.[10] A recent study showed a significant increase in BMI in adolescents with mothers working nonstandard work schedules, a reality in the work condition of mothers who belong to minority groups. These results indicate the importance of the association between maternal work schedules and adolescent weight increase, particularly in those 13 and 14 years of age.[11] Overall, these findings urgently argue for appropriate primary and secondary prevention programs, modified for the language, cultural, and medical needs of ethnic minorities.[12]

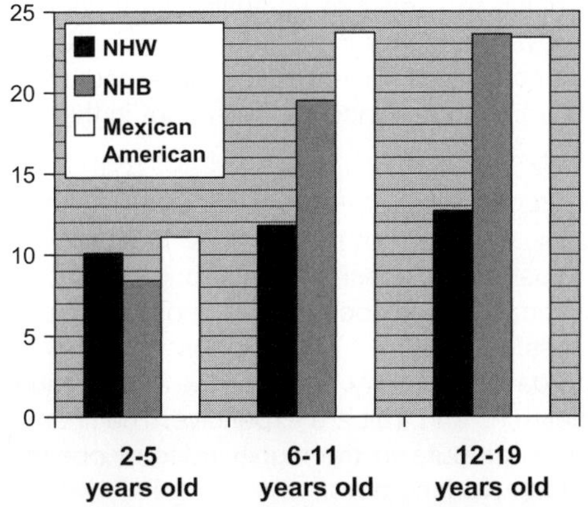

Fig. 2. Prevalence of overweight (BMI at 95th percentile or higher) in children and adolescents by race and ethnicity. NHB, non-Hispanic black; NHW, non-Hispanic white.

Although there is growing need to modify these behaviors in the population at large, the need is greatest among minorities and low-socioeconomic-status youth, particularly because of the overwhelmingly increased prevalence of obesity among minority groups.

Genetics may also play a role. It is not clear whether young people of different ethnic backgrounds differ in their adaptive mechanisms to obesity-related insulin resistance. In obese children and adolescents, mechanisms of adaptation to obesity-related insulin resistance are similar across ethnic groups. The greater early insulin response needed to maintain glucose tolerance in young people of ethnic minorities may partially explain their greater tendency to develop type 2 diabetes mellitus.[13] Asthma has proven to be a risk factor for obesity in children and adolescents. Considering the higher prevalence of asthma in minority populations, this disease process may be an independent risk factor to develop obesity in children from minority groups.[14]

THE PSYCHOSOCIAL PERSPECTIVE

Several factors may increase overweight risk among racial and ethnic minorities. Psychosocial disorders are known to affect obesity through central nervous system dysfunction, and these mechanisms are now being researched extensively. Efforts are underway to articulate environmental, psychosocial, and biological conditions that may predispose the development and maintenance of obesity. There is increasing evidence that adverse childhood experiences, such as childhood abuse, may be implicated in the development of obesity. This was demonstrated in a prospective, longitudinal study that tracked body mass across the development of childhood, through adolescence, and into young adulthood of abused and not abused female subjects.[15] There is additional evidence that associates psychosocial factors as a predictor for those who are at increased risk of developing the metabolic syndrome. This proves that psychosocial factors play a causal role in the events leading to the development of the metabolic condition.[16]

Immigrants, an essential component of the minority melting pot, face a significant number of factors in their adjustment and adaptation to the American "way of life." Although immigrants new to developed countries may be more vulnerable to the obesogenic environment, we lack established and effective strategies and interventions that specifically target their specific needs (eg, changes in dietary habits in the new country). These factors include the unavoidable clash of cultural values, the stresses and fears of the unknown in a mist of unfamiliar surroundings, language barriers, communication issues, and a higher incidence of anxiety and depressive disorders. These factors are suspected to be linked to the increased prevalence of weight gain and obesity that immigrants experience as they adapt in the United States and other industrialized countries.

THE SOCIOECONOMIC DETERMINANT

In the United States in particular, obesity has a strong socioeconomic etiological relationship. It seems related to limited social and economic resources and may be linked to disparities in access to healthy foods. Foods enriched in refined sugars and unhealthy fats are affordable and tasty, whereas the recommended lean meats, whole grains, and fresh vegetables and fruit are expensive. The financial disparity in access to healthier diets may contribute to the higher rates of obesity and diabetes found among minorities and the working poor.[17]

Environmental conditions that promote high-caloric content foods and impede the setting for regular physical activity are major contributors to the epidemic of obesity.

Societal determinants and strong environmental influences encourage overeating and sedentary behavior, yet the management of overweight and obesity conditions is often viewed as a personal responsibility. Past epidemiologic research studies have identified a single constant in the obesity equation. Obesity has been linked repeatedly to consumption of low-priced foods. The fact that energy-dense foods (megajoules/kilogram) cost less per megajoule than do nutrient-dense foods means that energy-dense diets are not only cheaper but may be preferentially selected by the lower-income consumer. In other words, the low cost of dietary energy (dollars/megajoule), rather than specific food, beverage, or macronutrient choices, may be the main predictor of population weight gain.[18] Neighborhoods where minorities typically live have more fast food restaurants and fewer vendors of quality foods than do predominantly wealthier neighborhoods. Physical activity is negated by unsafe streets, dilapidated parks, and lack of facilities.

There is evidence that, on average, immigrants are substantially less likely to be obese or overweight upon arrival to the adoptive country. These measures converge slowly to native-born levels, but there is marked variation by the ethnicity of the immigrant. Since changes in weight will reflect choices with respect to diet and activity, the extent to which overweight and obesity rates change with years in the new country may reflect the extent to which immigrants interact with, or are influenced by, members of their ethnic group who reside in the same area. For members of most ethnic minority groups, there is strong evidence that ethnic-group social network effects exert a quantitatively important influence on the incidence of being overweight and obese. With additional years in the adoptive country, these factors may temper the process of adjustment to the new culture lifestyle norms that may be driving excess weight gain.[19]

IMPLICATIONS FOR ACCESS AND QUALITY OF HEALTH CARE

It has been clearly established that the prevalence and severity of obesity are growing rapidly, along with obesity-related comorbidities and mortality. Given the increased health risks associated with obesity, it is vital that obese individuals have adequate access to, and make consistent use of, medical care services. Assuming obese people have access to medical care that is comparable to that for nonobese individuals, one would expect to observe greater use of medical services among those who are obese.

Minority groups that tend to have disproportionately high prevalence of obesity have reduced access to care, but it is not clear whether or not obese individuals have the same access to health care as do nonobese individuals. When looking at access and utilization of health care services, obesity has been consistently linked with greater rates of utilization and increased health care expenditures. Both the increased use and cost appear to be largely a function of treating obesity-associated comorbidities, such as diabetes and hypertension. It is probable that obesity is associated with both greater use and cost of medical care, but this relationship between obesity and access to medical care needs to be further studied.[20] Obese individuals are at higher risk of receiving poorer health care prevention and interventions. In spite of obesity increasing cancer risk, one study proved obesity to be associated with decreased Pap smear screening.[21] Small-scale surveys indicate that obese women delay or avoid cancer screening even more so than do nonobese women. In relationship to an increased BMI, white women were more likely to delay their Clinical breast examinations in comparison to nonwhite women. Thus, weight may be an important correlate of cancer screening behavior.[22] Further interventional studies are needed to determine barriers and effective interventions to improve screening in obese minority women.

Considering dental health, obesity status has its implications. As the incidence of obesity increases, it is likely that obese patients will present for dental services in greater numbers in the future. The implications of obesity on bone metabolism, craniofacial growth, and pubertal growth must be assessed in treating obese patients needing dental services, particularly orthodontic services. Dental health care professionals facing these issues should focus on relevant interventions concerning obesity with regard to dental care and orthodontic therapy.[23]

THE INFLUENCE OF GENETIC MAKEUP

Although related to greater caloric intake and lesser caloric utilization, obesity is not just an imbalance of energy input and expenditure. Clinical evidence and epidemiologic data clearly show that weight control is more complex than was expected by this simple equation. It is now known that common variants in genes play critical roles in determining susceptibility to the exposure to toxins and other environmental threats. For instance, neurologic research has proven that both addiction and obesity patients have similarities in their deficiency of dopamine receptors, a very provocative finding. Several relevant gene variants are present in most ethnic populations, but the frequency of their expression varies significantly, granting individuals or ethnic groups a greater susceptibility to particular environmental influences. Such findings are consistent with prior observations that showed how an individual can inherit the genetic predisposition to develop a disease but will do so only when exposed to the environmental factors that may trigger the disease process. The implication of this relationship has great importance when analyzing minority health determinants.

The genetic makeup of minority individuals does not differ significantly from everyone else's genetic pool. Nevertheless, minority individuals are exposed to different working and living conditions. These environments are known to have higher levels of multiple carcinogens or other toxic substances known to interact with susceptibility genes and potentially to cause disease. In addition, specific ethnic groups contributing to the minority group may see higher incidence of susceptible genes in their genetic makeup, placing them in a vulnerable and susceptible position relative to the adverse effects of the environmental threats they encounter in their daily lives. Most of the knowledge accrued related to the health effects of environmental threats is derived from studies of single environmental agents. We now know that environmental contributions to health disparities are not from isolated single factors but from multiple environmental agents. These multiple exposures to environmental risk factors may have the potential of accumulating or interacting synergistically, and the deleterious end results need further investigation.

One could extrapolate that much of the minority communities' disease burden could potentially be reduced through better environmental protection practices, especially in minority communities. Of the many implications of polymorphisms and frequency variations in the genetic makeup of minority individuals, none is more urgent than the choice of drugs in therapy. Using such knowledge, randomized trials have identified race-specific drug response differences between individuals of Caucasian origin and those of Asian, Hispanic, or African origin.[24]

INTERVENTION STRATEGIES

Traditional approaches to treating overweight and obese adults by focusing on individual weight loss have not been effective in reducing the increased rate of obesity in the general population. Recent research has identified critical factors that, if they accumulate and interact during an individual's life span, may put a person at risk for obesity. These factors include rapid weight gain in infancy and childhood, early puberty, and excessive weight gain in pregnancy. Based on this research, a lifecycle perspective can be used to develop comprehensive interventions that address the multiple determinants of obesity. Because obesity tracks across generations, it is essential to adopt effective obesity prevention measures now to prevent even higher rates of obesity in future generations.

In addressing the variety of health concerns raised by obesity, it is imperative that we look toward risk factor reduction. Intuitively targeting risk factors would appear to be an obvious solution to the problem of obesity in minorities. However, reports suggested that this approach may be faced with challenges due to the lack of scientific research involving minorities. The prevalence of risk factors differs considerably in minority populations. In people of African descent, "premature" coronary death and the level of some risk factors, particularly obesity and blood pressure, are found to be higher than those in whites. Some Hispanics have a higher triglyceride level, lower HDL, and increased incidence of diabetes in comparison to that in their white counterparts. With few exceptions, minorities have not been included in clinical trials in sufficient numbers to determine whether there is a significant benefit from current interventions aimed at risk factor reduction. There is no question that prevalence of key risk factors differs among minority groups. Risk factor intervention should be pursued in minority groups but with the understanding that clinical trials have not ruled out the possibility of qualitative or quantitative differences in response rates among different groups.[25]

Many diet-related chronic diseases take a disproportionate toll among members of ethnic and racial minorities. Research shows that the prevalence of diabetes, hypertension, cancer, and heart disease is higher among various ethnic groups compared with that in whites. Although somewhat different from what is encouraged by the Dietary Guidelines for Americans, abundant evidence has shown that regular exercise combined with diets lower in fat and richer in plant products is associated with reduced risk of these chronic conditions. Although ineffective dietary guidelines potentially put all Americans at unnecessary risk, this is particularly true for those groups hardest hit by chronic disease.[26]

There is an urgent need to identify areas for appropriate intervention, assess need for program development, and research priorities to implement developed best practice recommendations for minorities of all ages. Further research is required to understand the various strategies in which interventions are delivered and in which conditions they prove to be effective. There is a critical need for the development of consistent indicators to ensure that comparisons of program outcomes can be made to better inform best practice.[4]

Several studies have looked at BMI differences among various ethnic groups, and several attempts have been made to determine the factors that may contribute to these differences. Interestingly, adolescent food habits and physical activity have been found to be related to gender and ethnicity but not to socioeconomic factors. BMI has proven to be associated with ethnicity, gender, and food habits, but no significant relationship has been established with socioeconomic factors or physical activity. All studies have demonstrated the need to consider ethnicity, in addition to gender, when studying BMI and associated factors among obese adolescents.[27] Additionally, physical characteristics, nutrient intake, physical activity level, and body image have been demonstrated as different among Caucasian, African American, and Hispanic adolescents, once again emphasizing the importance of interventions that target improving health-related variables among minority populations.[28]

Cultural and linguistic emphasis is of great importance when designing interventions. A study designed to assess the impact of a culturally proficient dietary and physical activity intervention on changes in BMI, conducted between September 1999 and June 2002 in 12 Head Start preschool programs in Chicago, Illinois, proved effective in reducing subsequent increases in BMI in preschool children. This represents a promising approach to prevention of overweight among minority children in the preschool years.[29]

Dietetic professionals can reduce individual risks by providing nutritional services that support appropriate weight gain in pregnancy, childhood, and adulthood. Physicians should advocate for policies in communities, schools, and worksites that support breastfeeding, ensure access to health-promoting foods, and provide opportunities to be physically active.[30] Physicians should actively engage in the promotion of a healthier and more physically active lifestyle. This message should reach the executive levels in all industries and should be emphasized to policymakers who can advocate this need. Every participant must contribute to creating opportunities that will better the health of all Americans and ethnic minorities in particular.[31]

Parents of obese and overweight children are well positioned to drastically influence the eating habits of their children. Important aspects of the home environment include education, limited television viewing, and other parental behaviors that may contribute to childhood obesity. These factors should be assessed as potential targeted interventions.[9] Signed behavioral contracts committing to self-monitor eating and exercising patterns are a possible strategy. It has been proven that children whose parents self-monitor eating and exercise behavior were much more likely to consistently succeed at weight reduction and weight control. Self-monitoring is a cornerstone of successful weight control even for morbidly obese, low-income minority individuals. Targeting consistent self-monitoring among high-risk weight controllers and their parents should be just as important as it is for more affluent and less overweight adolescents.[32]

Medical societies and public health agencies, including departments of public health, have proposed the use of menu-board labeling of caloric content as a strategy to prevent overeating and the risk of obesity. Although valuable, the effectiveness of menu-board labeling is counteracted by a phenomenon called *optimistic bias.*[33] Through this psychological mechanism, individuals rationalize their choices and believe they have a lower risk for an adverse event than the average population. Optimistic bias will prompt individuals to avoid making good food choices. Physicians should educate their patients on the importance of menu and caloric reading and interpretation and make patients understand the concept of optimistic bias and how to prevent its influence on the food choices they make.

Interestingly, when comparing obesity treatments with addiction interventions, significant differences are found. Obesity treatments do not consider different levels or type and intensity of care, and they lack a multidimensional approach. To overcome these limitations, a biopsychosocial approach in which the genetic influence is matched by psychosocial issues and mental health issues may be advantageous. This approach may influence the treatment options, by focusing both on the lessons coming from actual addiction treatment and the opportunities offered by virtual reality.[34] Obesity control efforts must be shifted away from individual-level approaches toward population-based approaches that address socioeconomic, behavioral, and environmental factors. Unfortunately, studies have not addressed particular populations, including ethnic minority groups. Several studies have inspected the effectiveness of population-based interventions targeting vulnerable populations but have fallen short of including sufficient samples to permit ethnic-specific analyses. Further research is needed to develop sound strategies to engage and retain members of minority groups in these interventions. These population-based strategies are as important, if not more essential, as proposed interventions directed to individual weight loss, regular physical activity, or healthier eating habits. Physicians are the best-equipped advocates to develop and support policy directed at increasing the visibility and budget priority of these interventions.[35]

Comprehensive policy approaches that emphasize behavioral nutrition and that take into account the economics of food choice are in great need. Encouraging low-income households to consume more costly foods as the main goal in combating obesity is economically not feasible, and, therefore, it is a counterproductive approach to improving the health of vulnerable populations. It is not an effective strategy for advancement of public health.[17]

Health disparities are a significant public health problem that cannot simply be solved using established funding mechanisms and priority setting. The current emphasis on basic and clinical research, which excludes public health and the social sciences, does not provide the interdisciplinary research teams necessary to address such a complex problem as health disparities. A radical change in the socioeconomic status of a specific population is a huge undertaking. However, improving their health status via strategies that integrate current genetic knowledge with other established factors could potentially greatly improve the health outcome of minority populations. Social, environmental, and genetic scientists must work in interdisciplinary ways to develop more accurate and relevant ways to address the health of disadvantaged communities.[36]

SUMMARY

It is evident that obesity is a growing medical concern worldwide. It is an epidemic that has dramatically affected the health of all Americans. Minorities carry excess burden of cardiovascular risk factors, particularly high blood pressure, diabetes, obesity, physical inactivity, and psychosocial stress. Further research describing the link between obesity and atherosclerosis and heart disease is much needed.

Cultural factors in symptom recognition and health care–seeking behavior are of great importance. The complex interplay of the factors involved in health care disparities should be considered. Economic factors influencing access to health care, including prevention, diagnosis, and treatment, are also essential parts of the equation. Psychosocial stress, ethnic and racial disparities, and frustration, leading to suboptimal interactions with the health care system, must be considered as important as the genetics and predisposition to obesity. These are fundamental factors in the causation and, therefore, the potential solution for ethnic disparities in obesity prevention and treatment.

The associations of obesity with gender, age, ethnicity, and socioeconomic status are complex and dynamic. Related population-based programs and policies are needed.

Childhood overweight continues to increase rapidly in the United States, particularly among African Americans and Hispanics. Culturally competent treatment strategies as well as other policy interventions are required to increase physical activity and encourage healthy eating patterns among children.[8] In considering all possible causes of population differences in obesity prevalence, which include biologic susceptibility, decreased regular physical activity, availability of effective treatment modalities, cultural factors, and behavioral determinants, it is important to understand how cultural elements and environmental conditions play a significant role in the increased prevalence of obesity in minority groups in the United States.

Without question, inequities in exposure to health education, quality health care, and adequate environmental conditions are in part responsible for the increased rate of obesity and its consequences in minority populations. Interventions for the prevention and treatment of obesity in minority populations must address these inequities. The growing interest in obesity in minority populations reflects an awareness of the high prevalence of obesity among minority groups as well as a generally increased interest in minority health. We should continue to pay close attention to obesity as it occurs in and affects ethnic minorities, which includes African Americans, Hispanic Americans, Asian and Pacific Islander Americans, American Indians and Alaska Natives, and Native Hawaiians in the United States.

REFERENCES

1. Flegal KM, Carroll MD, Ogden CL, et al. Prevalence and trends in obesity among US adults, 1999–2000. JAMA 2002;288(14):1723–7.
2. Foreyt JP, Poston WS 2nd. Obesity: a never-ending cycle? Int J Fertil Womens Med 1998;43(2):111–6.
3. Buchowski MS, Sun M. Nutrition in minority elders: current problems and future directions. J Health Care Poor Underserved 1996;7(3):184–209.
4. Lobstein T. Comment: preventing child obesity—an art and science. Obes Rev 2006;7(Suppl 1):1–5.
5. Will B, Zeeb H, Baune BT. Overweight and obesity at school entry among migrant and German children: a cross-sectional study. BMC Public Health 2005;5:45.
6. Goran MI. Metabolic precursors and effects of obesity in children: a decade of progress, 1990–1999. Am J Clin Nutr 2001;73(2):158–71.
7. Ogden CL, Flegal KM, Carroll MD, et al. Prevalence and trends in overweight among US children and adolescents, 1999–2000. JAMA 2002;288(14):1728–32.
8. Strauss RS, Pollack HA. Epidemic increase in childhood overweight, 1986–1998. JAMA 2001;286(22):2845–8.
9. Kumanyika S, Grier S. Targeting interventions for ethnic minority and low-income populations. Future Child 2006;16(1):187–207.
10. Shaibi GQ, Ball GD, Goran MI. Aerobic fitness among Caucasian, African-American, and Latino youth. Ethn Dis 2006;16(1):120–5.
11. Miller DP, Han WJ. Maternal nonstandard work schedules and adolescent overweight. Am J Public Health 2008;98(8):1495–502.
12. Sundquist J, Winkleby MA, Pudaric S. Cardiovascular disease risk factors among older black, Mexican-American, and white women and men: an analysis of NHANES III, 1988–1994. Third National Health and Nutrition Examination Survey. J Am Geriatr Soc 2001;49(2):109–16.
13. Weiss R, Dziura JD, Burgert TS, et al. Ethnic differences in beta cell adaptation to insulin resistance in obese children and adolescents. Diabetologia 2006;49(3): 571–9. Epub 2006 Feb 3.
14. Gennuso J, Epstein LH, Paluch RA, et al. The relationship between asthma and obesity in urban minority children and adolescents. Arch Pediatr Adolesc Med 1998;152(12):1197–200.
15. Noll JG, Zeller MH, Trickett PK, et al. Obesity risk for female victims of childhood sexual abuse: a prospective study. Pediatrics 2007;120(1):e61–7.
16. Raikkonen K, Matthews KA, Kuller LH. Depressive symptoms and stressful life events predict metabolic syndrome among middle-aged women: a comparison

of World Health Organization, Adult Treatment Panel III, and International Diabetes Foundation definitions. Diabetes Care 2007;30(4):872–7.
17. Drewnowski A, Darmon N. Food choices and diet costs: an economic analysis. J Nutr 2005;135(4):900–4.
18. Drewnowski A. The real contribution of added sugars and fats to obesity. Epidemiol Rev 2007;29:160–71.
19. McDonald JT, Kennedy S. Is migration to Canada associated with unhealthy weight gain? Overweight and obesity among Canada's immigrants. Soc Sci Med 2005;61(12):2469–81.
20. Fontaine KR, Bartlett SJ. Access and use of medical care among obese persons. Obes Res 2000;8(5):403–6.
21. Ferrante JM, Chen PH, Jacobs A. Breast and cervical cancer screening in obese minority women. J Womens Health (Larchmt) 2006;15(5):531–41.
22. Fontaine KR, Heo M, Allison DB. Body weight and cancer screening among women. J Womens Health Gend Based Med 2001;10(5):463–70.
23. Neeley WW 2nd, Gonzales DA. Obesity in adolescence: implications in orthodontic treatment. Am J Orthod Dentofacial Orthop 2007;131(5):581–8.
24. Moyer VA, Klein JD, Ockene JK, et al. Screening for overweight in children and adolescents: where is the evidence? a commentary by the childhood obesity working group of the US Preventive Services Task Force. Pediatrics 2006; 116(1):235–8.
25. LaRosa JC, Brown CD. Cardiovascular risk factors in minorities. Am J Med 2007; 120(3):e15 and e17; author reply e19.
26. Bertron P, Barnard ND, Mills M. Racial bias in federal nutrition policy, Part II: weak guidelines take a disproportionate toll. J Natl Med Assoc 1999;91(4):201–8.
27. Kumar BN, Holmboe-Ottesen G, Lien N, et al. Ethnic differences in body mass index and associated factors of adolescents from minorities in Oslo, Norway: a cross-sectional study. Public Health Nutr 2004;7(8):999–1008.
28. Perry AC, Rosenblatt EB, Wang X. Physical, behavioral, and body image characteristics in a tri-racial group of adolescent girls. Obes Res 2004;12(10):1670–9.
29. Fitzgibbon ML, Stolley MR, Schiffer L, et al. Two-year follow-up results for Hip-Hop to Health Jr.: a randomized controlled trial for overweight prevention in preschool minority children. J Pediatr 2005;146(5):586–90.
30. Johnson DB, Gerstein DE, Evans AE, et al. Preventing obesity: a life cycle perspective. J Am Diet Assoc 2006;106(1):97–102.
31. Shephard RJ. The value of physical fitness in preventive medicine. Ciba Found Symp 1985;110:164–82.
32. Kirschenbaum DS, Germann JN, Rich BH. Treatment of morbid obesity in low-income adolescents: effects of parental self-monitoring. Obes Res 2005;13(9): 1527–9.
33. Miles S, Scaife V. Optimistic bias and food. Nutr Res Rev 2003;16(1):3–19.
34. Riva G, Bachetta M, Cesa G, et al. Is severe obesity a form of addiction? Rationale, clinical approach, and controlled clinical trial. Cyberpsychol Behav 2006; 9(4):457–79.
35. Yancey AK, Kumanyika SK, Ponce NA, et al. Population-based interventions engaging communities of color in healthy eating and active living: a review. Prev Chronic Dis 2004;1(1):18.
36. Olden K, White SL. Health-related disparities: influence of environmental factors. Med Clin North Am 2005;89(4):721–38.

Overweight and Obesity in Children and Adolescents

Nathan F. Bradford, MD

KEYWORDS

• Obesity • Overweight • Body mass index

Becoming obese or overweight is a leading threat to the health of children and adolescents worldwide. The prevalence of obesity and overweight has doubled and even tripled in certain age groups. Most overweight children become overweight adults.[1] Given the adverse effects seen on health from obesity in adults, it is clear that childhood obesity is setting the stage for tremendous individual and societal health costs in the future. Much research has been undertaken to understand the causes of obesity with a view to prevention. Finally, along with recommendations for office evaluation and treatment of childhood obesity and overweight are presented.

DEFINITIONS

In 1997, an Expert Committee convened by the US Department of Health and Human Services set recommendations on the evaluation and treatment of childhood and adolescent obesity. These recommendations have since been revised in 2007 by another Expert Committee convened by the American Medical Association and the Centers for Disease Control and Prevention (CDC) with representatives from 15 national health care organizations, with the further task of defining this problem. This Expert Committee recommends a yearly check for obesity/overweight in adolescents and children by measuring the body mass index (BMI) (kg/m^2). The BMI correlates with excess body fat as well as with health risks.[2–4] BMI is plotted on charts released by the CDC in 2000, which rank weight by height, age, and sex (**Figs. 1–3**). The term "overweight" replaced the term "at risk for overweight" for a BMI greater than or equal to the 85th percentile, whereas the term "obesity" replaced "overweight" for those with BMI greater than or equal to the 95th percentile or BMI of 30 kg/m^2 (the adult cutoff for obesity). BMI varies with age such that there is a decrease until about 6 years, the nadir, after which BMI gradually rises with age, a phenomenon known as the "adiposity rebound."[5] A third category of "severe obesity" refers to BMI greater than or equal to the 99th percentile; children in this category are at an even greater risk of morbidity and mortality.[6]

AnMed Family Medicine Residency Program, 2000 East Greenville Street, Suite 3600, Anderson, SC 29621, USA
E-mail address: nathan.bradford@anmedhealth.org

Prim Care Clin Office Pract 36 (2009) 319–339
doi:10.1016/j.pop.2009.01.002 **primarycare.theclinics.com**

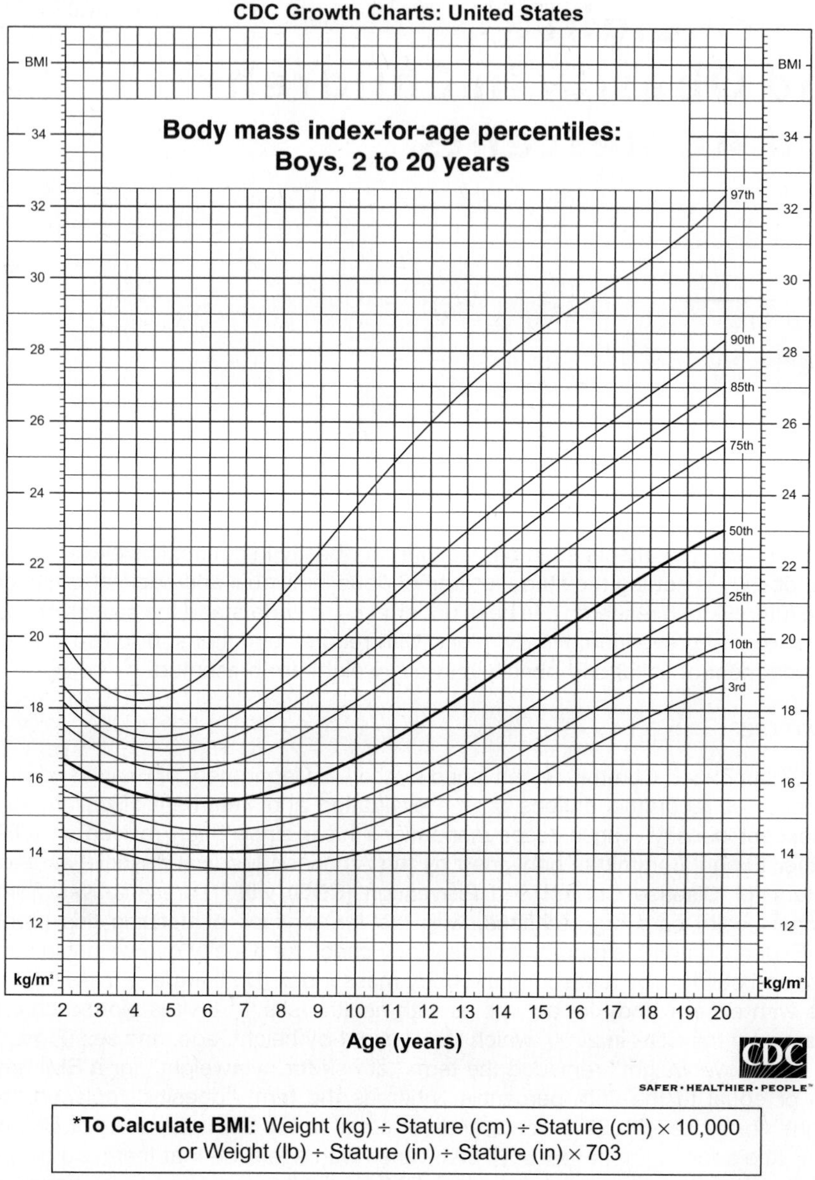

Fig. 1. BMI for boys aged 2 to 20 y. (*From* Centers for Disease Control and Prevention. CDC Growth Charts, United States. Available at: http://www.cdc.gov/nchs/about/major/nhanes/growthcharts/charts.htm.)

EPIDEMIOLOGY

The CDC collects data on the US population every few years with the National Health and Nutrition Examination Survey (NHANES). From the 1960s to 1980, the prevalence of obesity in children remained stable, but from the 1976-to-1980 period to the 2003-to-2004 period, the prevalence of obesity (defined as BMI $\geq$ the 95th percentile)

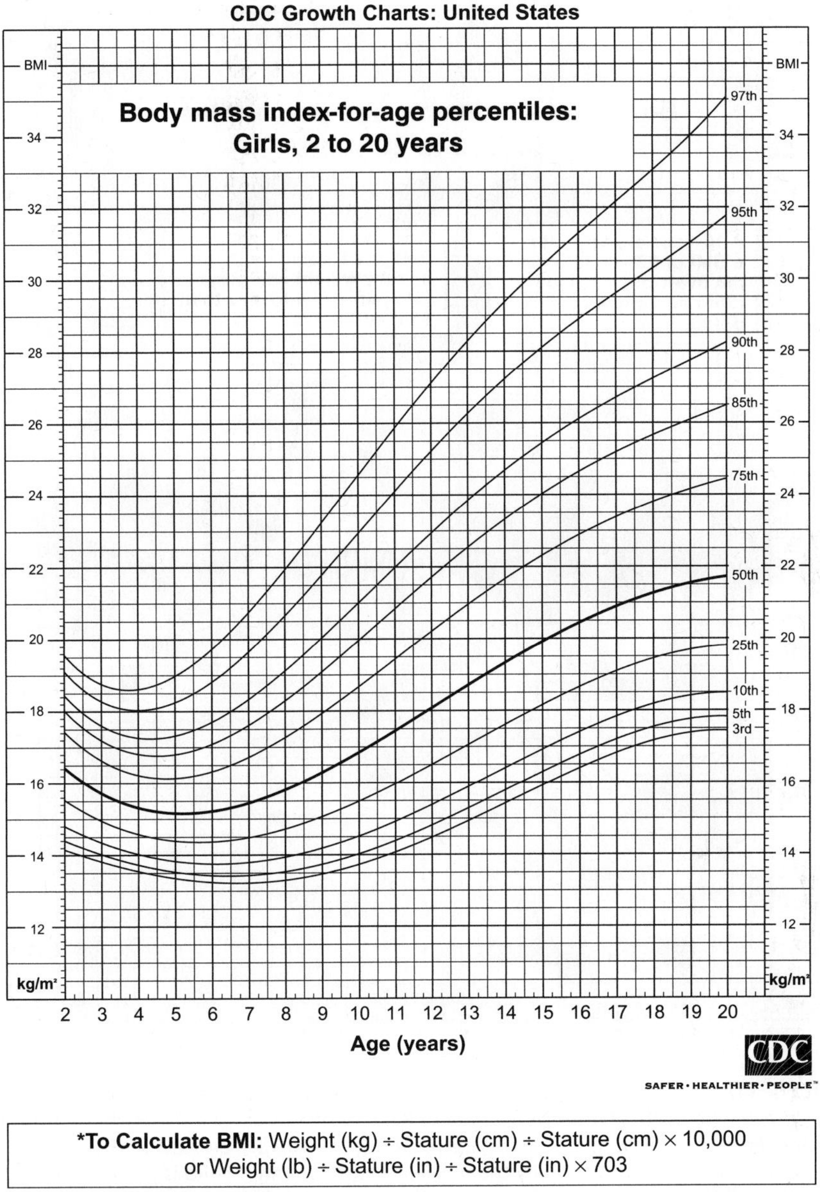

Fig. 2. BMI for girls aged 2 to 20 y. (*From* Centers for Disease Control and Prevention. CDC Growth Charts, United States. Available at: http://www.cdc.gov/nchs/about/major/nhanes/growthcharts/charts.htm.)

increased dramatically in all age groups (**Table 1**). The prevalence of obesity doubled in 2- to 5-year-olds from 7.2% to 13.9%. In 6- to 11-year-olds, the prevalence went from 11% to 19%, and in 12- to 19-year-olds from 11% to 17%.[7] Overall, in the 2003-to-2004 survey, 17% of children and adolescents were obese.[8]

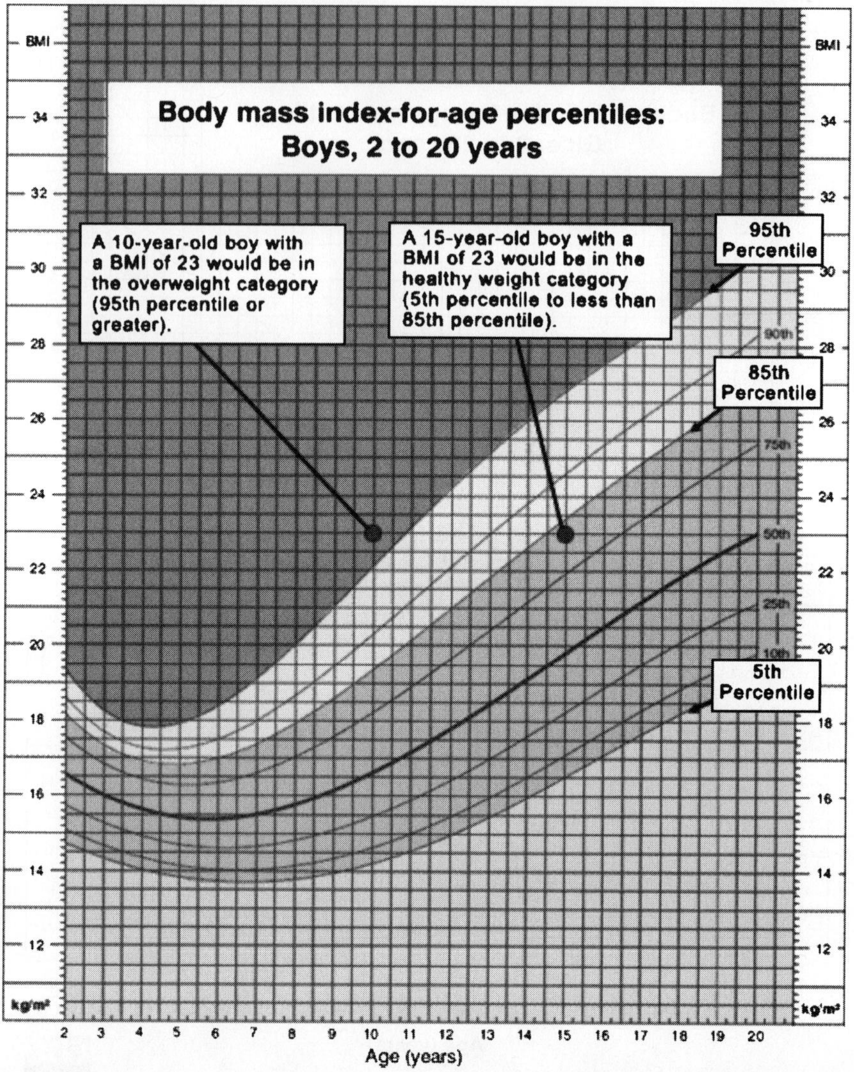

Fig. 3. The BMI number has different meanings by age. An example of a 10-y-old boy and a 15-y-old boy who both have a BMI-for-age of 23. For a 10-y-old, this BMI is obese but for the 15-y-old, this is normal weight. The children of different ages are plotted on the same growth chart to illustrate a point. Normally the measurement for only 1 child is plotted on a growth chart. (*From* Centers for Disease Control and Prevention. Healthy Weight. Available at: http://www.cdc.gov/healthyweight/assessing/bmi/childrens_bmi/about_childrens_bmi.html.)

ETIOLOGY

The etiology of overweight and obesity has traditionally been understood in a biopsychosocial framework, in which multiple factors overlap (**Fig. 4**).[9]

Genetic and Biologic Factors

Hundreds of genes and genetic markers have been linked with obesity. Currently, researchers are focusing on the leptin gene mutation (leptin reduces appetite),

Table 1
Prevalence of obesity (BMI ≥ the 95th percentile) among children and adolescents aged 2 to 19 years, for selected years 1963–1965 through 1999–2004

Age (y)[a]	NHANES 1963–1965 1966–1970[b]	NHANES 1971–1974	NHANES 1976–1980	NHANES 1988–1994	NHANES 1999–2000	NHANES 2001–2002	NHANES 2003–2004
2–5	—	5	5	7.2	10.3	10.6	13.9
6–11	4.2	4	6.5	11.3	15.1	16.3	18.8
12–19	4.6	6.1	5	10.5	14.8	16.7	17.4

[a] Excludes pregnant women starting with 1971–1974. Pregnancy status not available for 1963–1965 and 1966–1970.
[b] Data for 1963–1965 are for children aged 6–11 y; data for 1966–1970 are for adolescents aged 12–17 y not 12–19 y.
From Centers for Disease Control and Prevention. Overweight and obesity. Available at: http://www.cdc.gov/nccdphp/dnpa/obesity/childhood/prevalence.htm.

melanocortin 4 receptor mutation (hormone acting on receptor increases energy output and decreases appetite), and hormones such as ghrelin. (Ghrelin is made in the fundus of the stomach; it rises before a meal, signaling hunger, and falls after a meal, signaling satiety).[9–16] Analogues to hormones such as peptide YY are being developed to try to inhibit appetite by acting on the gut to delay emptying and on the brain to decrease appetite.[17–19] Another peptide, amylin, is secreted with insulin and acts similarly to peptide YY.[20,21] On the whole, however, genetic causation for obesity is thought to involve a combination of genetic mutations, not just one.[9,22]

Effective treatments arising from these discoveries are not yet ready for "prime time." Leptin supplements are available but have not benefited patients with leptin mutations.[23] An analogue to amylin has the ability to lower blood sugar and cause

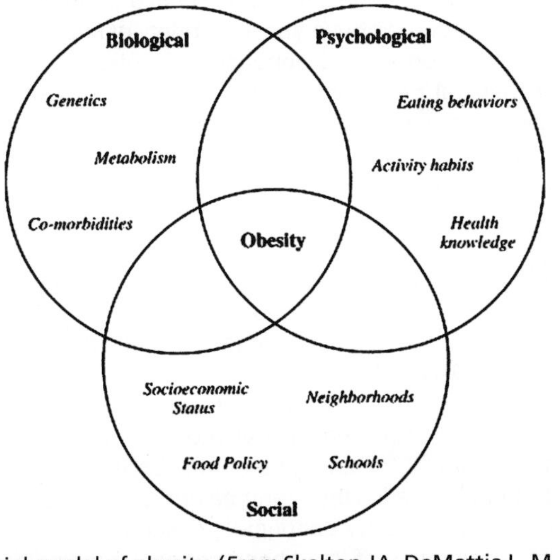

Fig. 4. Biopsychosocial model of obesity. (*From* Skelton JA, DeMattia L, Miller L, et al. Obesity and its therapy: from genes to community action. Pediatr Clin North Am 2006;53:4.)

weight loss.[24] One recent finding, rimonabant, causes weight loss as well as improves cardiac factors.[25] Rimonabant is an appetite suppressant, which blocks the cannabinoid-1 receptor found in the CNS and in peripheral tissues.[26]

Many familial syndromes include or lead to obesity including Prader-Willi, muscular dystrophy, Turner syndrome, and hyperinsulinism. Specific gene mutations are thought to be responsible for a small proportion of obesity, in the range of 5% to 10%. However, more broadly, genetic factors contribute to a third of obesity. Twins reared apart show concordance in their weights, illustrating the importance of genetics over environment.[27] Furthermore, twins show similar adiposity responses to caloric excess and deprivation.[28] Genetics influence resting energy expenditure, with white children consuming more calories at rest than African American children.

In the United States, obesity is most common in Hispanic youth, less common in African American youth, and least common in Caucasian youth. Historically, this phenomenon has been attributed to a supposed "thrifty gene" associated with certain races.[29] Early puberty increases the risk of adult obesity. Parental obesity increases the risk for young obese children to become obese adults.[30]

Another way in which genetics influences obesity is that eating behaviors appear to be inherited.[9] Faith and coauthors have found genetic links for food preferences, the ability to taste fat, and eating disorders.[31–33] However, it seems that the family environment is at least as strong in shaping a child's eating preferences.[34]

Other possible biologic mechanisms for the development of obesity include infection. Adenovirus infection in mice has been associated with obesity.[35–37] Additionally, the adipocyte itself has endocrine capabilities, in that it produces and secretes inflammatory markers, which have been dubbed "adipokines." These have given credence to the idea that obesity is an inflammatory state. As further support for this theory, white cells are found in adipose tissue.[38–40]

Medical Conditions and Treatments

Endocrine disorders such as hypothyroidism, hypercortisolism, or Cushing's syndrome, or growth hormone deficiency can all have short stature, slow growth velocity, and of course obesity. Some rare endocrine causes include insulinomas and pseudohypoparathyroidism. Children who survive brain damage, brain tumors, or brain irradiation often become obese due to a variety of factors including decreased physical activity and alterations in neuroendocrine function.[41,42]

Medications and medical treatments can lead to obesity. The medications most commonly associated with obesity are corticosteroids, progestins, valproate, cyproheptadine, and mirtazapine. The atypical antipsychotics can lead not only to weight gain but also to diabetes and hyperlipidemia.

Prenatal to Infancy

Environmental factors have long been known to be associated with obesity and overweight, starting with pregnancy. Babies born small for gestational age (SGA), with small head circumferences, short lengths, or to a diabetic mother are all at increased risk of overweight.[43–45] SGA babies who are given high-calorie diets are at increased risk for obesity.[46] A theory to explain this states that there are critical periods in growth and development during which nutritional or environmental factors increase the risk of obesity and hyperinsulinism.[47–49] Perhaps the most important of these periods is the intrauterine period, and it appears that early caloric deprivation signals the fetus to alter its genetic makeup (the "thrifty genotype") in such a way as to hold on to calories.[50] Perhaps another example of this phenomenon is the finding that teens whose mothers smoked during pregnancy are more likely to be obese.[51]

The presence and duration of breastfeeding have been shown to protect against obesity. Addition of solids or juice to the infant's diet, as opposed to exclusive breastfeeding, is a risk factor for later obesity.[52,53] When a child is overweight, the risk of adult obesity depends on the age at which the child becomes overweight. Overweight children less than 3 years old are less likely to become overweight adults than older children. In fact, the older a child is when he or she becomes obese, the more likely that child will be obese as an adult, and girls tend to have persistent obesity more than boys do.[30,54,55] The normal age at which children increase their BMI is around 5 to 7 years; this is called the adiposity rebound. When the adiposity rebound occurs earlier, the risk for obesity increases. Furthermore, rapid weight gain during certain critical periods seems to increase the risk of obesity persistence to later life.[56]

Parental Factors

At all ages, the presence of parental obesity at least doubles the risk of a child's being overweight as an adult. Out of all risk factors for obesity, parental obesity, especially in the mother, seems to be the strongest. Furthermore, parental practices in feeding children can lead to obesity. Too much control over a child's food choices leads to obesity due to the child learning not to respond to hunger or satiety impulses.[57] Dieting itself in young children is linked to more loss of control or binge eating.

Sedentary and Sleep Habits

One of the best-studied environmental factors influencing childhood obesity is television (TV) viewing. The amount of time spent watching TV directly correlates with the risk of childhood and adult obesity.[58] A recent study also shows a strong direct association between TV viewing and fast food eating.[59] The association of video games with obesity is less robust.[60,61] Proposed explanations for the correlation between obesity and "screen time" (total viewing including computer, video games, and TV) include less energy expenditure, a slower metabolic rate, worse eating habits, and snacking.[62] Furthermore, on an average day of watching TV, a child is likely to view 12 to 30 food commercials, which has been found to increase children's consumption of fast food and sugar-sweetened drinks and to decrease their consumption of fruits and vegetables.[62,63]

Lack of exercise is highly correlated with obesity. In a 2001 study, Nesmith[64] found that only 50% of young Americans aged 12 to 21 years regularly participate in rigorous physical activity, and 25% report no physical activity. Barriers to exercise include living in unsafe neighborhoods. A parent's perception that the neighborhood is unsafe is more important in whether the child goes out to play than how safe the neighborhood actually is in terms of crime data.[65] Furthermore, children are 4 times more likely to be obese in the first grade if the parent perceives the neighborhood as unsafe.[66] Children in general also tend to decrease the amount of time spent in exercise between childhood and adolescence.[67]

Another lifestyle factor is sleep deprivation, which has been associated with obesity in both children and adults.[68–70] In a study of Japanese children aged 6 to 7 years, those sleeping less than 8 hours nightly were nearly 3 times as likely to be obese as those sleeping 10 or more hours nightly.[70] Lack of sleep increases ghrelin levels and decreases leptin levels, both of which can lead to obesity.[71,72]

Dietary Factors

Several dietary factors have been linked to obesity, including TV viewing causing increased snacking, ingestion of fast food, lack of family meal times, meal times spent watching TV, and daily consumption of sweetened drinks. Sugar-sweetened drinks increase the risk of obesity.[73,74] Obese children tend to skip breakfast and consume less calcium.[75] In a study of fifth graders, children who skipped breakfast were 1.5 times as likely to be overweight.[76] Eating meals together as a family 3 to 4 times a week significantly decreased overweight.[77] In developed countries, there is a plethora of high-calorie, convenient meals, snacks, and drinks, which make it very easy to consume excessive calories without being aware of it. A typical fast food meal has around 2000 calories and contains 84 g of fat. A third of American children eat a fast food meal each day,[5] and fast food eating increases during the transition from adolescence to young adulthood.[59] In general, in the United States, one consumes up to 50% more calories when eating out than those consumed when eating at home. Snacking is another behavior that contributes to obesity. In a study of 21,236 children 2 to 18 years between 1977 and 1996, it was found that snacking increased by 24% to 36%, accounting for 25% of energy intake by 1996.[78]

A comparison of causal factors for obesity separated by what can and cannot be modified is represented in **Table 2**.

COMORBID CONDITIONS

Diabetes Mellitus

Type 2 diabetes mellitus, impaired fasting glucose (IFG), impaired glucose tolerance (IGT), and insulin resistance are some of the serious complications of obesity. Diabetes mellitus is defined as a fasting glucose greater than or equal to 126; IFG, a fasting glucose 101 to 125; and IGT, a blood glucose between 140 and 200 mg/dL after an oral glucose challenge. Insulin resistance is an inappropriate blood glucose elevation in response to elevation in insulin level and is highly correlated with truncal obesity measured by waist circumference. In one study of obese children and adolescents, 25% of children and 21% of adolescents had IGT, whereas 4% of adolescents had asymptomatic type 2 diabetes.[79] Children and adolescents with type 2 diabetes may have subtle presentations, lacking the well-known symptoms of type 1 diabetes, polyuria, polyphagia, and polydipsia. Therefore, screening is paramount in obese and overweight children.

Table 2
Modifiable and nonmodifiable factors in obesity

Modifiable	Nonmodifiable
Prenatal factors	Family history of obesity (particularly parental)
Maternal smoking	Syndromes that cause obesity
Intrauterine growth problems	Genetic mutations
Infancy	Medical conditions
Not breastfeeding	Early adiposity rebound
Diet	Hispanic or African American descent
Poor diet (fast food, snacking, sweetened beverages)	
Family eating behaviors	
Parental control	
Not eating breakfast	
Sedentary behaviors	
Lack of exercise	
Increased time spent watching TV	
Lack of sleep	
Medications	

In the SEARCH for Diabetes in Youth study, a multicenter study of diabetes in children and adolescents conducted by the CDC and the National Institute of Diabetes and Digestive and Kidney Diseases, 92% of children and adolescents newly diagnosed with type 2 diabetes mellitus have at least 2 of the following: elevated triglycerides, low high-density lipoprotein (HDL), elevated blood pressure, or elevated waist circumference.[80]

Hypertension

The risk of hypertension increases in overweight and obese children and adolescents. It may be due to sodium retention, increased sympathetic tone, or increased angiotensin system activity.[81] Obesity is also associated with increased left ventricular mass in children.[82] Obese children and adolescents have a 3-fold increased risk of developing hypertension.[83] Increased waist circumference is independently associated with hypertension.[84]

Hyperlipidemia

Hyperlipidemia is associated with obesity in children, in the pattern of increased triglycerides and low-density lipoprotein and decreased HDL. The accumulation of fat in the abdomen correlates more strongly with hyperlipidemia than with its accumulation in the hips or a more general increase in BMI.[85]

Metabolic Syndrome

For many years, an association between various cardiovascular risk factors (insulin resistance, obesity, hypertension, and hyperlipidemia) has been noted, known as Syndrome X or the metabolic syndrome. Given the fact that atherosclerosis has been known to start in young children, it is reasonable to study this syndrome in children. Many sets of criteria for the metabolic syndrome are known, and the Third Report of the National Cholesterol Education Program Adult Treatment Panel defines it as the presence of an elevation of any 3 of the following: blood sugar, waist circumference, lipids, or blood pressure. Using these factors and the NHANES III (1988–1994), an overall prevalence of metabolic syndrome in all adolescents is 4.2%.[86] Taking adolescents with BMI greater than or equal to the 95th percentile, 28.7% have 3 risk factors, meeting the definition for metabolic syndrome.[87] The Pediatric Metabolic Syndrome Working Group using data from the NHANES 1999–2002 demonstrated an increasing prevalence of metabolic syndrome with increasing BMI.[88]

Polycystic Ovarian Syndrome or Hyperandrogenism

Central obesity in adolescent girls and women is associated not only with excessive insulin production and resistance but also with excessive production of androgens. These in turn lead to the features common to polycystic ovarian syndrome (PCOS): male pattern hair distribution, acne, striae, and dysfunctional uterine bleeding. PCOS occurs in at least 8% of young women 18 to 25 years of age.

Obstructive Sleep Apnea

Obstructive sleep apnea (OSA) is part of a spectrum of disorders known as sleep-disordered breathing, which also includes snoring and daytime alveolar hypoventilation. Diagnosis is by an overnight sleep study, and historically, OSA has been related to hypertrophy of the tonsils and adenoids in children and adolescents. However, a second and more common form of OSA is emerging, which is 4 to 6 times more common in obese children.[89,90] The prevalence of some type of sleep-disordered breathing is thought to be near 50% in obese children.[91] The manifestations in children are similar to those in adults, with resulting elevated blood pressure, left ventricular remodeling, daytime sleepiness, hyperactivity, restlessness, inattentiveness, and aggression. Both the cardiovascular and the neuropsychological consequences improve in children with treatment of OSA.

Orthopedic Complications

Overweight and obese children are at increased risk for several orthopedic conditions. Complaints of pain and impaired mobility are more common in overweight and obese children and adolescents. Slipped capital femoral epiphysis is more common in overweight boys between ages 9 and 16 years and presents with hip or referred knee pain. These patients will have more pain with walking. Diagnosis is with frog-leg radiographic views of the hips. Blount's disease, or tibia vara, is bowing of the tibias and is more common in the overweight child older than 8 years. Radiographic studies in anterior-posterior views of the affected knee diagnose the condition. Referral to an orthopedic surgeon is indicated for either of these conditions. Obese and overweight children are more likely to report fractures, musculoskeletal discomfort, impaired mobility, and lower extremity malalignment.[92] Unfortunately, these problems likely discourage children from physical activity, thus worsening the underlying problem of obesity.

Mental Health

Many associations between obesity and psychological factors exist, but causality has not been established. Obese children as young as 5 years are aware of their obesity, with the result being decreased self-esteem.[93] Girls are more prone to self-esteem problems than boys.[94] Children perceive obesity as less desirable than physical deformities and disease. They tend to associate obesity with laziness, greed, and lower intelligence quotient.[95] However, parental acceptance of their obesity bolsters their self-esteem. About 20% to 40% of severely obese adolescents suffer from loss of control eating, and these individuals are more likely to suffer from anxiety, depression, and low self-esteem.[96,97] Nearly half of severely obese adolescents report moderate to severe depressive symptoms, and a third report anxiety.[98]

More information about mental health and obesity in all populations is in the section "Mental Health."

Neurologic Disorders

Being overweight is one of the causes of pseudotumor cerebri at any age. Children and adolescents with this condition, also known as benign intracranial hypertension, present with headache, decreased vision, papilledema, and isolated sixth nerve palsy. This condition is more prevalent even with a 10% increase in body weight more than normal, and there is an increasing prevalence with increasing BMI.[99]

More information about comorbidities of obesity in all populations is in the section "Cardiovascular Disease and other Comorbidities."

EVALUATION

The evaluation of an obese or overweight child should proceed along the lines of the chronic illness model. Although this may be difficult, because some insurance carriers may not reimburse for obesity treatment, the American Academy of Pediatrics (AAP) has a coding fact sheet available at: www.aap.org/healthtopics/overweight.cfm.[100,101] First, a family history should be obtained to identify inherited causes for obesity as well as tendencies toward exogenous obesity. The history should include other medical illnesses, particularly any medical treatments undertaken. Psychosocial factors, such as eating patterns and physical activity, should be discussed. A history of binge eating or loss of control eating should lead to an investigation of eating disorders. Any psychological or psychiatric comorbidities should be explored. Next, history should be obtained regarding any symptoms of weight-related problems, such as frequent urination, abnormal thirst, or history of hyperglycemia, to look for diabetes; abdominal pain or nausea for nonalcohol fatty liver disease; joint pain for orthopedic concerns; and breathing problems and exercise tolerance to evaluate pulmonary abilities and hypoventilation.

After BMI is plotted on the CDC growth chart by age and sex, blood pressure should be obtained at each health maintenance visit. The blood pressure reading is compared on the National Heart, Lung, and Blood Institute table, which plots blood pressure against age, gender, and height percentile, and hypertension is diagnosed by 3 readings more than the 95th percentile for systolic or diastolic blood pressure.

The physical examination focuses on weight-related findings. These include acanthosis nigricans or dark velvety skin around the neck, often associated with diabetes and striae, indicating rapid weight gain or hypercortisolism. The striae of rapid weight gain are flesh-colored, whereas the striae seen in Cushing's syndrome are violaceous in color. Musculoskeletal examination focuses on bowing of the legs and muscle mass. An endocrine examination looks for abnormal distribution of fat, such as the "buffalo hump" or "moon facies" seen in Cushing's syndrome. Excessive hair growth raises the possibility of PCOS, especially in a male pattern. The examination focuses on any dysmorphology, Tanner staging, height, and edema, looking for evidence of a genetic disorder. Obesity makes Tanner staging more difficult; adipose tissue can look like breast development, whereas pigmented, erectile areolae are characteristic of true breast development. A suprapubic fat pad should be manually deflected to see the true size of the penis. Generally, the obese child matures faster than the nonobese child.

At 10 years, an overweight child with 2 risk factors should begin having blood drawn every other year for fasting glucose, lipid panel, aspartate aminotransferase (AST), and alanine aminotransferase (ALT) (**Table 3**).[102] Risk factors are a family history of type 2 diabetes mellitus; being of Native American, Alaskan, or African American descent; or having other signs associated with hyperinsulism, such as acanthosis nigricans, hyperandrogenism, or cardiovascular risk factors. ALT or AST levels greater than 60 should prompt further evaluation directed by a specialist. For obese children, the same laboratory tests should be performed even in the absence of risk factors.[103] Glucose tolerance testing, although more sensitive in identifying diabetes, is more costly and, therefore, not recommended. Thyroid testing, although frequently performed, is generally unnecessary in an overweight child with normal linear growth velocity and no symptoms of hypothyroidism.

Table 3
Recommendations for laboratory evaluation of children 10 y and older

BMI ≥85th percentile with 2 risk factors (African American, Native American, or Hispanic, family history of type 2 diabetes mellitus, signs of hyperinsulinism)	Every other year: lipids, glucose, AST, ALT
BMI > 95th percentile	Every other year: lipids, glucose, AST, ALT

PREVENTION AND TREATMENT

Obesity in childhood not only causes high morbidity but also predisposes to adult obesity.[1] Treatment of childhood and adolescent obesity is very difficult. Therefore, it is paramount to enact prevention strategies at every age, beginning with the perinatal period. Unfortunately, no firm evidence exists yet that any 1 strategy results in a lower BMI long term.[1] Since large size for gestational age, often associated with gestational diabetes mellitus, often leads to obesity,[1] careful control of blood sugar during pregnancy is warranted. Conversely, small size for gestational age is associated with childhood obesity, so careful attention to prenatal factors that impact placental sufficiency is advised.[1] Careful control of maternal weight before conception as well as maternal weight gain during pregnancy may also help mitigate childhood obesity.

Breastfeeding should be encouraged, because it is inversely correlated with obesity. In a meta-analysis of 69,000 infants, breastfeeding was found to have a small but significant effect on preventing obesity.[104] Although no critical time period has been determined, it appears that several months of exclusive breastfeeding gives the best protection against obesity.[105] Therefore, introduction of solids and juices should be postponed.

For toddlers and school-aged children, the 2007 Expert Committee recommends counseling parents as part of their "Prevention Plus" strategy to eat less fast food, eat meals together at set meal times, follow healthy diets, and turn off the TV during meals (**Box 1**).[101] Other recommendations from the Expert Committee include eating foods high in calcium, fiber, and macronutrients. Parents should disregard packaging sizes on prepackaged foods in favor of portion sizes that are more appropriate for children. Sugar-sweetened drinks including fruit juice should be eliminated from the diet; whole fruits are a better source of vitamins and minerals. Eating out should be curtailed as well. Parents should be encouraged to not only direct children to exercise for 60 minutes each day but also to be physically active themselves. In family-based weight management programs, change in parental behavior is correlated with success in the child.[106] Family-based behavioral therapy has been found to lead to weight loss in children. The important ingredient seems to be the inclusion of the parents in the therapy.[107] Because children with obese parents are more likely to become obese themselves, counseling should include and be directed at obese parents too.

Box 1
The 2007 Expert Committee recommendations known as "Prevention Plus"

Limit consumption of sugar-sweetened beverages

Follow the United States Department of Agriculture (USDA) dietary recommendations (9 servings of fruits and vegetables a day). See the USDA Web site (www.mypyramid.gov) for age-appropriate recommendations on specific amounts of fruits and vegetables

Follow the AAP recommendations that total daily "screen time" (which includes TV, computer, and video games) is limited to 2 h/d

Eat breakfast daily

Eat meals together as a family

Decrease eating out at restaurants, especially fast food restaurants

Follow USDA recommendations on portion sizes instead of packaging portion sizes

Caloric reduction is the *sine qua non* of weight loss. Low-carbohydrate, high-protein diets, such as the Atkins diet, have become popular for adolescents. A 12-week study comparing a low-carbohydrate diet to a low-fat diet in 30 obese adolescents (mean age, 14; mean BMI, 35) showed a 5-kg advantage in weight loss for the low-carbohydrate diet.[108] Another study showed that a low-carbohydrate diet was superior to a low-fat diet in achieving weight loss.[109] Since a high-concentrated carbohydrate meal results in a greater insulin surge than a meal higher in fat or protein, these findings would make sense. Moreover, fiber intake reduces the risk of type 2 diabetes mellitus and cardiovascular disease.[110] However, there is not enough evidence to recommend any particular diet other than a reduced-calorie diet with less than 30% of calories as fat.[111] Although many different diets are proposed for children and adolescents, the bottom line is that weight loss will occur if less calories are consumed.

For the older child and adolescent, evidence suggests that there are benefits from counseling not only the parents but also the child's peer group as well; in the Eating Among Teens study, the intake of fast food in males was inversely correlated with peer group support for eating healthy foods.[112] This could be done through school clinics, other teaching opportunities in schools, and in group medical visits.

Exercise has several benefits for the overweight child. It influences fasting insulin levels more strongly than obesity does.[113] One study of obese children shows that 40 minutes a day of exercise produces a 5% weight loss as well as a reduction in insulin and triglyceride levels, apart from diet.[114] A meta-analysis of evidence-based exercise recommendations found that 60 minutes a day of exercise that is age appropriate and enjoyable would result in health benefits, including weight loss.[115] However, a Cochrane Review of trials focusing on physical activity alone showed marginal results,[116] and studies that employed both diet and exercise to treat obesity were also disappointing.[116]

Barriers to exercise include living in unsafe neighborhoods. When a parent feels that it is too dangerous to send the child out to play, it is recommended that the physician not try to convince the parent otherwise but to offer suggestions for indoor play, such as using an indoor exercise mat or jumping rope or exercising at a local fitness club with the parent participating, thus serving as a role model. In the Walking School Bus program (www.walkingschoolbus.org or www.cdc.gov/nccdphp/dnpa/kidswalk), parents or adult volunteers walk with the children to school.[65]

Once the child or adolescent is overweight, the primary care provider and office should engage motivational techniques to encourage the patient and the family to lose weight. Historically, counseling provided to parents regarding childhood behavior has been directive, presenting information with advice, known as "anticipatory guidance." More recently "Motivational Interviewing" (MI), developed in the addiction field, has been used with some success in dealing with child and adolescent overweight.[117] Pediatricians and dieticians using MI with overweight children and an obese parent have been successful in producing significant weight loss.[117] MI is a way of eliciting change from an individual not by persuasion or arguing but by encouraging him or her to draw on his or her own aspirations and desires, in effect allowing the patient to do the psychological work.[118] In MI, the parent and patient are assessed not only for motivation to change but also for awareness of the problem; this is helpful, because often parents of overweight and obese children are not aware of the problem.[119]

A simple way of accomplishing MI is to use the DARES mnemonic, which stands for Develop Discrepancy, Avoid Argumentation, Roll with Resistance, Express Empathy, and Support Self-Efficacy.[118] Briefly, the first step is to "Express Empathy," which encompasses acceptance of the patient's problems and concerns without passing judgment. Secondly, to "Develop Discrepancy," the clinician helps the patient see how his or her behavior is not consistent with his goals. Thirdly, "Avoid Argumentation" expresses the truth that arguing with patients does not usually lead to change. Fourth, "Roll with Resistance" refers to the counselor's not becoming defensive or angry with a patient's refusal to change but to redirect the patient's momentum into some avenue of change. Finally, "Support Self-efficacy" is to let the patient see the underlying assumption that the patient has the inner resources and strength needed to change.[118] Examples of MI are listed in **Box 2**.

For the child or adolescent who does not lose weight with the above interventions, the next step is "Structured Weight Management," an intensive approach characterized by more structure and oversight. The child and family are under the care of a dietician to provide specific and structured dietary changes. A more structured exercise program ideally includes the use of daily logs and the input of a physical or exercise therapist. The patient is seen in the office monthly, possibly for group sessions, and the office staff gives more intensive MI. Family counseling may help with weight loss by producing changes in family eating patterns or resolving conflict.[101]

If the above are ineffective, the next step is a more intensive program dubbed "Comprehensive Multidisciplinary Intervention" in which the child is seen in specialty offices on an even more frequent basis, possibly weekly. The multidisciplinary team includes a behavioral counselor or some other professional with experience in childhood obesity in addition to the primary care physician, dietician, exercise specialist, and/or a community program for obese children.[101]

To be a candidate for oral medications or surgery, the child or adolescent should have passed into the multidisciplinary stage. One medication that has been FDA approved for use in adolescents 16 years and older is sibutramine, a norepinephrine and serotonin reuptake inhibitor. It has been shown to enhance weight loss in adolescents by an additional 3 kg when compared with that with exercise and diet

Box 2
Examples of MI using DARES

Mother frequently relies on fast food to feed her family in the evenings:

It sounds as if it is really hard in the evenings, getting everyone home and fed. (Express empathy.)

You obviously are doing a great job keeping Sarah healthy…she always gets her shots on time, and you bring her in whenever she is sick….But do you think that her weight might cause some health problems later on for her? (Develop discrepancy.)

Do you think she would be happier in the future if she were a little slimmer? (Avoid argumentation.)

Can you think of any way you can help her lose a little weight? (Support self-efficacy.)

Mother keeps children in front of the TV as a babysitter:

It sounds like it is really hectic at your house—no wonder it's a relief for the kids to be occupied for a while! (Express empathy.)

Do you think the TV watching might be contributing to John's weight gain? (Develop discrepancy.)

I wonder if he snacks more when he is watching TV? (Avoid argumentation.)

Are there other situations in which he *does* tend to snack? (Roll with resistance.)

Have you come up with any good ideas for helping him cut down on his snacks? (Support self-efficacy.)

Box 3
Criteria for gastric banding or bypass in adolescents and children

BMI $\geq$40 kg/m^2 with a medical condition or BMI $\geq$50 kg/m^2

Emotional, physical, and cognitive maturity

Weight loss efforts in a behavior-based treatment program for 6 mo

alone.[120,121] Orlistat is a drug that is not systemically absorbed and acts to block absorption of fats from the diet by inhibiting intestinal lipase. It is approved for adolescents 12 years and older and provides some benefit.[122] Both of these drugs have been studied only in conjunction with diet and exercise. Metformin causes very modest weight loss in adults but is not approved for this purpose, because the weight loss is not significant enough. However, it may be beneficial in the child or adolescent who has developed or who is at risk for type 2 diabetes mellitus[123] or has hyperinsulinism and infertility associated with polycystic ovary syndrome.[124] Medications for obesity in children are considered to be of little value, with unclear risks. Notably, although many adolescents use dietary supplements, no evidence exists to support their use.[125] More in-depth information about pharmacologic treatment of obesity is at "Pharmacotherapies."

Bariatric surgery is becoming more common for the severely obese adolescent. When combined with psychological and nutritional support, surgery can produce significant and lasting weight loss.[126] Criteria for gastric banding or bypass in children and adolescents are in **Box 3**.[127]

SUMMARY

Child and adolescent obesity is becoming more prevalent. Many exciting discoveries exist in the causes—environmental, behavioral, and genetic—which provide fruitful possibilities for prevention and treatment. All children should be screened for overweight/obesity with a yearly BMI. The evaluation of the overweight or obese pediatric patient should proceed as with any other chronic medical problem, with a careful history, physical examination, and targeted blood chemistry evaluation. Any evidence of comorbidities should prompt further evaluation directed by findings in history and physical examination. Treatment of overweight and obesity is based on BMI and on previous treatment attempts and success. Although the initial treatment is always diet and exercise, some medical and surgical therapies show promise in the pediatric population. Other exciting possibilities based on genetic and biologic etiologies of obesity are on the horizon.

REFERENCES

1. Guo SS, Wu W, Chumlea WC, et al. Predicting overweight and obesity in adulthood from body mass index values in childhood and adolescence. Am J Clin Nutr 2002;76:653–8.
2. Pietrobelli A, Faith MS, Allison DB, et al. Body mass index as a measure of adiposity among children and adolescents: a validation study. J Pediatr 1998; 132:204–10.
3. Mei Z, Grummer-Strawn LM, Pietrobelli A, et al. Validity of body mass index compared with other body-composition screening indexes for the assessment of body fatness in children and adolescents. Am J Clin Nutr 2002;75:978–85.

4. Freedman DS, Khan LK, Dietz WH, et al. Relationship of childhood obesity to coronary heart disease risk factors in adulthood: the Bogalusa Heart Study. Pediatrics 2001;108:712–8.
5. Skelton JA, Rudolph CD. Overweight and obesity. In: Kliegman RM, Behrman RE, Jenson HB, et al, editors. Nelson textbook of pediatrics. 18th edition. Philadelphia: Saunders; 2007.
6. Freedman DS, Mei Z, Srinivasan SR, et al. Cardiovascular risk factors and excess adiposity among overweight children and adolescents: the Bogalusa Heart Study. J Pediatr 2007;150:12–7.
7. Prevalence of Overweight Among Children and Adolescents: United States, 2003–2004. National Center for Health Statistics, CDC website. Available at: www.cdc.gov/nchs/products/pubs/pubd/hestats/overweight/overwght_chld_03.htm. Accessed November 12, 2008.
8. Ogden C, Carroll MD, Curtin LR, et al. Prevalence of overweight and obesity in the United States, 1999–2004. JAMA 2006;295:1549–55.
9. Skelton JA, DeMattia L, Miller L, et al. Therapy: from genes to community action. Pediatr Clin North Am 2006;53(4):777–94.
10. Zhang Y, Proenca R, Maffei M, et al. Positional cloning of the mouse obese gene and its human homologue. Nature 1994;372:425–32.
11. Tschop M, Weyer C, Tataranni PA, et al. Circulating ghrelin levels are decreased in human obesity. Diabetes 2001;50:707–9.
12. Druce MR, Wren AM, Park AJ, et al. Ghrelin increases food intake in obese as well as lean subjects. Int J Obes 2005;29:1130–6.
13. Vaisse C, Clement K, Guy-Grand B, et al. A frameshift mutation in human MC4R is associated with a dominant form of obesity. Nat Genet 1998;20:113–4.
14. Farooqi IS, Keogh JM, Yeo GS, et al. Clinical spectrum of obesity and mutations in the melanocortin 4 receptor gene. N Engl J Med 2003;348:1085–95.
15. Cummings DE, Overduin J. Gastrological regulation of food intake. J Clin Invest 2007;117(1):13–23.
16. Inui A, Asakawa A, Bowers C, et al. Gastric bypass: ghrelin, appetite, and gastric motility: the emerging role of the stomach as an endocrine organ. FASEB J 2004;18(3):439–56.
17. Batterham RL, Cohen MA, Ellis SM, et al. Inhibition of food intake in obese subjects by peptide YY3-36. N Engl J Med 2003;349:941–8.
18. Batterham RL, Cowley MA, Small CJ, et al. Gut hormone PYY(3-36) physiologically inhibits food intake. Nature 2002;418:650–4.
19. Boggiano MM, Chandler PC, Oswald KD, et al. PYY3-36 as an anti-obesity drug target. Obes Rev 2005;6:307–22.
20. Reidelberger RD, Kelsey L, Heimann D. Effects of amylin-related peptides on food intake, meal patterns, and gastric emptying in rats. Am J Physiol Regul Integr Comp Physiol 2002;282:R1395–404.
21. Reidelberger RD, Haver AC, Arnelo U, et al. Amylin receptor blockade stimulates food intake in rats. Am J Physiol Regul Integr Comp Physiol 2004;287: R458–574.
22. Clement K. Genetics of human obesity. Proc Nutr Soc 2005;64:133–43.
23. Bell-Anderson KS, Bryson JM. Leptin as a potential treatment for obesity: progress to date. Treat Endocrinol 2004;3:11–8.
24. Schmitz O, Brock B, Rungby J. Amylin agonists: a novel approach in the treatment of diabetes. Diabetes 2004;53:S233–8.
25. Pi-Sunyer FX, Aronne LJ, Heshmati HM, et al. Group RI-NAS. Effect of rimonabant, a cannabinoid-1 receptor blocker, on weight and cardiometabolic risk

factors in overweight or obese patients: RIO-North America: a randomized controlled trial. JAMA 2006;295:761–75.
26. Cota D, Marsicano G, Tschop M, et al. The endogenous cannabinoid system affects energy balance via central orexigenic drive and peripheral lipogenesis. J Clin Invest 2003;112:423–31.
27. Maes HH, Neale MC, Eaves LJ. Genetic and environmental factors in relative body weight and human adiposity. Behav Genet 1997;27:325–51.
28. Perusse L, Bouchard C. Gene-diet interactions in obesity. Am J Clin Nutr 2000; 72:1285S–90S.
29. Neel JV. Diabetes mellitus: a "thrifty" genotype rendered detrimental by "progress"? Am J Hum Genet 1962;14:353–62.
30. Whitaker RC, Wriht JA, Pepe MS, et al. Predicting obesity in young adulthood from childhood and parental obesity. N Engl J Med 1997;337:869–73.
31. Faith MS, Johnson SL, Allison DB. Putting the behavior into the behavior genetics of obesity. Behav Genet 1997;27:423–39.
32. Faith MS, Keller KL, Johnson SL, et al. Familial aggregation of energy intake in children. Am J Clin Nutr 2004;79:844–50.
33. Faith MS. Development and modification of child food preferences and eating patterns: behavior genetics strategies. Int J Obes 2005;29:549–66.
34. Wardle J, Guthrie C, Sanderson S, et al. Food and activity preferences in children of lean and obese parents. Int J Obes 2001;25(7):971–7.
35. Dhurandhar NV, Kulkarni P, Ajinkya SM, et al. Effect of adenovirus infection on adiposity in chicken. Vet Microbiol 1992;31:101–7.
36. Dhurandhar NV, Whigham LD, Abbott DH, et al. Human adenovirus Ad-36 promotes weight gain in male rhesus and marmoset monkeys. J Nutr 2002;132:3155–60.
37. Dhurandhar NV, Israel BA, Kolesar JM, et al. Increased adiposity in animals due to a human virus. Int J Obes Relat Metab Disord 2000;24:989–96.
38. Fantuzzi G. Adipose tissue, adipokines, and inflammation. J Allergy Clin Immunol 2005;115:911–9.
39. Hutley L, Prins JB. Fat as an endocrine organ: relationship to the metabolic syndrome. Am J med Sci 2005;330:280–9.
40. Bouloumie A, Curat CA, Sengenes C, et al. Role of macrophage tissue infiltration in metabolic diseases. Curr Opin Clin Nutr Metab Care 2005;8:347–54.
41. Lustig RH, Post SR, Srivannaboon K, et al. Risk factors for the development of obesity in children surviving brain tumors. J Clin Endocrinol Metab 2003;88(2):611–6.
42. Tiosano D, Eisentein I, Militianu D, et al. 11 Beta-hydroxysteroid dehydrogenase activity in hypothalamic obesity. J Clin Endocrinol Metab 2003;88:379–84.
43. Hediger ML, Overpeck MD, McGlynn A, et al. Growth and fatness at three to six years of age of children born small-or large-for-gestational age. Pediatrics 1999; 104:e33 [abstract].
44. Cox JT, Phelan ST. Nutrition during pregnancy. Obstet Gynecol Clin North Am 2008;35(3):369–83, viii.
45. McMillen IC, MacLaughlin SM, Muhlhausler BS, et al. Developmental origins of adult health and disease: the role of periconceptional and foetal nutrition. Basic Clin Pharmacol Toxicol 2008;102(2):82–9.
46. Prentice AM, Goldberg GR. Energy adaptations in human pregnancy: limits and long-term consequences. Am J Clin Nutr 2000;71(Suppl 5):1226s–32s.
47. Huxley R, Owen CG, Whincup PH, et al. Is birth weight a risk factor for ischemic heart disease in later life? Am J Clin Nutr 2007;85:1244–50.
48. Barker DJ, Winter PD, Osmond C, et al. Weight in infancy and death from ischaemic heart disease. Lancet 1989;2:984–5.

49. Fernandez-Twinn DS, Ozanne SE. Mechanisms by which poor early growth programs type-2 diabetes, obesity and the metabolic syndrome. Physiol Behav 2006;88:234–43.
50. Candib LM. Obesity and diabetes in vulnerable populations: reflection on proximal and distal causes. Ann Fam Med 2007;5(6):547–56.
51. Al Mamun A, Lawlor DA, Alati R, et al. Does maternal smoking during pregnancy have a direct effect on future offspring obesity? evidence from a prospective birth cohort study. Am J Epidemiol 2006;164(4):317–25 [abstract].
52. Grummer-Strawn LM, Mei Z. Does breastfeeding protect against pediatric overweight? Analysis of longitudinal data from the Centers for Disease Control and Prevention Pediatric Nutrition Surveillance System. Pediatrics 2004;113:e81–6.
53. Victora CG, Barros F, Lima RC, et al. Anthropometry and body composition of 18 year old men according to duration of breast feeding: birth cohort study from Brazil. BMJ 2003;327:901.
54. Garn SM, LaVelle M. Two-decade follow-up of fatness in early childhood. Am J Dis Child 1985;139:181–5.
55. Garn SM, Cole PE. Do the obese remain obese and the lean remain lean? Am J Public Health 1980;70:351–3.
56. Monteiro PO, Victora CG. Rapid growth in infancy and childhood and obesity in later life—a systematic review. Obes Rev 2005;6:143–54.
57. Birch LL, Fisher JO. Development of eating behaviors among children and adolescents. Pediatrics 1998;101:539–49.
58. Neumark-Sztainer D, Story M. The Henry J. Kaiser Family Foundation. The role of media in childhood obesity. Available at: http://www.kff.org/entmedia/upload/32431_1.pdf. Accessed November 12, 2008.
59. Larson NI, et al. Fast food intake: longitudinal trends during the transition to young adulthood and correlates of intake. J Adolesc Health 43(1):79–86.
60. Stettler N, Signer TM, Suter PM. Electronic games and environmental factors associated with childhood obesity in Switzerland. Obes Res 2004;12:896–903.
61. Kautiainen S, Koivusilta L, Lintonen T, et al. Use of information and communication technology and prevalence of overweight and obesity among adolescents. Int J Obes (Lond) 2005;29:925–33.
62. Ludwig DS, Gortmaker SL. Programming obesity in childhood. Lancet 2004;364:226–7.
63. Coon KA, Tucker KL. Television and children's consumption patterns. A review of the literature. Minerva Pediatr 2002;54:423–36.
64. Nesmith JD. Type 2 diabetes mellitus in children and adolescents. Pediatr Rev 2001;22:147–52.
65. Lumeng JC, Appugliese D, Cabral HJ, et al. Neighborhood safety and overweight status in children. Arch Pediatr Adolesc Med 2006;160:25–31.
66. Matthieu J. Safe play and its effect on childhood obesity. J Am Diet Asssoc 2008;108(5):774–5.
67. Nader PR, Bradley RH, Houts RM, et al. Moderate-to-vigorous physical activity from ages 9 to 15 years. JAMA 2008;300(3):295–305.
68. Chaput JP, Tremblay A. Does short sleep duration favor abdominal adiposity in children? Int J Pediatr Obes 2007;2:188–91.
69. Flint J, Kothare SV, Zihlif M, et al. Association between inadequate sleep and insulin resistance in obese children. J Pediatr 2007;150:364–9.
70. Sekine M, Yamagami T, Handa K, et al. A dose-response relationship between short sleeping hours and childhood obesity: results of the Toyama Birth Cohort Study. Child Care Health Dev 2002;28:163–70.

71. Taheri S, Lin L, Austin D, et al. Short sleep duration is associated with reduced leptin, elevated ghrelin, and increased body mass index. PLoS Med 2004;1(3): e62.
72. Spiegel K, Tasali E, Penev P, et al. Brief communication: sleep curtailment in healthy young men is associated with decreased leptin levels, elevated ghrelin levels, and increased hunger and appetite. Ann Intern Med 2004;141: 846–50.
73. Ludwig DS, Peterson KE, Gortmaker SL. Relation between consumption of sugar-sweetened drinks and childhood obesity: a prospective, observational analysis. Lancet 2001;357:505–8.
74. Giammattei J, Blix G, Marshak HH, et al. Television watching and soft drink consumption: associations with obesity in 11- to 13-year-old schoolchildren. Arch Pediatr Adolesc Med 2003;157:882–6.
75. Heaney RP, Davies KM, Barger-Lux MJ. Calcium and weight: clinical studies. J Am Coll Nutr 2002;21:152S–5S.
76. Veugelers PJ, Fitzgerald AL. Prevalence of and risk factors for childhood overweight and obesity. CMAJ 2005;173:668–73.
77. Gortmaker SL, Must A, Perrin JM, et al. Social and economic consequences of overweight in adolescence and young adulthood. N Engl J Med 1993;329:1036 [abstract].
78. Jahns L, Siega-Riz AM, Popkin BM. The increasing prevalence of snacking among US children from 1977 to 1996. J Pediatr 2001;138(4):493–8.
79. Sinha R, Fisch G, Teague B, et al. Prevalence of impaired glucose tolerance among children and adolescents with marked obesity. N Engl J Med 2002; 346:802–10.
80. Rodriguez BL, Fujimoto WY, Mayer-Davis EJ, et al. Prevalence of cardiovascular risk factors in type 2 diabetes in children and adolescents: the SEARCH for Diabetes in Youth study. Diabetes Care 2006;29(8):1891–6.
81. Berkowitz C. Obesity in children. First Consult 2007;4 [online journal].
82. Hanevold C, Waller J, Daniels S, et al. The effects of obesity, gender, and ethnic group on left ventricular hypertrophy and geometry in hypertensive children: a collaborative study of the International Pediatric hypertension Association. Pediatrics 2004;113(2):328–33.
83. Sorof J, Daniels S. Obesity hypertension in children: a problem of epidemic proportions. Hypertension 2002;40:441–7.
84. Maffeis C, Pietrobelli A, Grezzani A, et al. Waist circumference and cardiovascular risk factors in prepubertal children. Obes Res 2001;9:179–87.
85. Caprio S, Hyman LD, McCarthy S, et al. Fat distribution and cardiovascular risk factors in obese adolescent girls: importance of the intraabdominal fat depot. Am J Clin Nutr 1996;64:12–7.
86. Goodman E, Daniels SR, Morrison JA, et al. Contrasting prevalence of and demographic disparities in the World Health Organization and National Cholesterol Education Program Adult Treatment Panel III definitions of metabolic syndrome among adolescents. J Pediatr 2004;145:445–51.
87. Cook S, Weitzman M, Auinger P, et al. Prevalence of a metabolic syndrome phenotype in adolescents: findings from the third National Health and Nutrition Examination Survey, 1988–94. Arch Pediatr Adolesc Med 2003;157:821–7.
88. Weiss R, Dziura J, Burgert TS, et al. Obesity and the metabolic syndrome in children and adolescents. N Engl J Med 2004;350:2362–74.
89. Dayyat E, Kheirandish-Gozal L, Gozal D. Childhood obstructive sleep apnea: one or two distinct disease entities? Sleep Med Clin 2007;2:433–44.

90. Young T, Peppard PE, Gottlieb DJ. Epidemiology of obstructive sleep apnea: a population health perspective. Am J Respir Crit Care Med 2002;165: 1217–39 [abstract].
91. Verhulst SL, Schrauwen N, Haentjens D, et al. Sleep-disordered breathing in overweight and obese children and adolescents: prevalence, characteristics and the role of fat distribution. Arch Dis Child 2007;92:205–8.
92. Taylor ED, Theim KR, Mirch MC, et al. Orthopedic complications of overweight in children and adolescents. Pediatrics 2006;117:2167–74.
93. Schwimmer JB, Burwinkle TM, Varni JW. Health-related quality of life of severely obese children and adolescents. JAMA 2003;289:1813–9.
94. Strauss RS, Pollack HA. Social marginalization of overweight children. Arch Pediatr Adolesc Med 2003;157:746–52.
95. Epstein LH, Roemmich JN, Raynor HA. Behavioral therapy in the treatment of pediatric obesity. Pediatr Clin North Am 2001;48:981–93.
96. Zametkin AJ, Zone CK, Klein HW, et al. Psychiatric aspects of child and adolescent obesity: a review of the past 10 years. J Am Acad Child Adolesc Psychiatry 2004;43:134–50.
97. Britz B, Siegfried W, Ziegler A, et al. Rates of psychiatric disorders in a clinical study group of adolescents with extreme obesity and in obese adolescents ascertained via a population based study. Int J Obes Relat Metab Disord 2000;24: 1707–14.
98. Falkner NH, Neumark-Sztainer D, Story M, et al. Social, educational, and psychological correlates of weight status in adolescents. Obes Res 2001;9:32–42.
99. Giuseffi V, Wall M, Siegel PZ, et al. Symptoms and disease associations in idiopathic intracranial hypertension (pseudotumor cerebri): a case-control study. Neurology 1991;41:239–44.
100. Story MT, Neumark-Stzainer DR, Sherwood NE, et al. Management of child and adolescent obesity: attitudes, barriers, skills, and training needs among health care professionals. Pediatrics 2002;110:210–4.
101. Barlow SE, et al. Expert Committee recommendations regarding the prevention, assessment, and treatment of child and adolescent overweight and obesity: summary report. Pediatrics 2007;120S:S164–92.
102. Gahagan S, Silverstein J. The Committee on Native American Child Health and Section on Endocrinology. Prevention and treatment of type 2 diabetes mellitus in children, with special emphasis on American Indian and Alaska Native children. Pediatrics 2003;112:e328.
103. American Diabetes Association. Type 2 diabetes in children and adolescents. Pediatrics 2000;105:671–80.
104. Arenz S, Ruckerl R, Koletzko B, et al. Breast-feeding and childhood obesity—a systematic review. Int J Obes Relat Metab Disord 2004;28:1247–56.
105. Bogen DL, Hanusa BH, Whitaker RC. The effect of breast-feeding with and without formula use on the risk of obesity at 4 years of age. Obes Res 2004; 12:1527–35 [abstract].
106. Wrotniak BH, Epstein LH, Paluch RA, et al. Parent weight change as a predictor of child weight change in family–based behavioral obesity treatment. Arch Pediatr Adolesc Med 2004;158:342–7.
107. Epstein LH, Valoski AM, Wing RR, et al. Ten-year follow-up of behavioral family-based treatment for obese children. JAMA 1990;264:2519–23.
108. Sondike SB, Copperman N, Jacobson MS. Effects of a low-carbohydrate diet on weight loss and cardiovascular risk factor in overweight adolescents. J Pediatr 2003;142:253–8.

109. Ebbeling CB, Leidig MM, Sinclair KB, et al. A reduced-glycemic load diet in the treatment of adolescent obesity. Arch Pediatr Adolesc Med 2003;157:773–9.
110. Slavin J. Why whole grains are protective: biological mechanisms. Proc Nutr Soc 2003;62:129–34.
111. Levine MJ. Low-carbohydrate diets: assessing the science and knowledge gaps, summary of an ILSI North America Workshop. J Am Diet Assoc 2006; 106(12):2086–94.
112. Neumark-Sztainer D, Wall M, Perry C, et al. Correlates of fruit and vegetable intake among adolescents: findings from Project EAT. Prev Med 2003;37(3): 198–203.
113. Allen DB, Nemeth BA, Clark RR, et al. Fitness is a stronger predictor of fasting insulin levels than fatness in overweight male middle school children. J Pediatr 2007;150(4):383–7.
114. Ferguson MA, Gutin B, Le NA, et al. Effects of exercise training and its cessation on components of the insulin resistance syndrome in obese children. Int J Obes Relat Metab Disord 1999;23:889–95.
115. Strong WB, Malina RM, Blimkie CJ, et al. Evidence based physical activity for school-age youth. J Pediatr 2005;146(6):732–7.
116. Summerbell CD, Waters E, Edmunds LD, et al. Interventions for preventing obesity in children. Cochrane Database Syst Rev 2005;(3):CD001871.
117. Schwartz R, Hamre R, Dietz WH, et al. Office-based motivational interviewing to prevent childhood obesity. Arch Pediatr Adolesc Med 2007;161:495–501.
118. Miller WR, Rollnick S. Motivational interviewing. New York: The Guilford Press; 1991. p. 55–63.
119. Rhee KE, De Lago CW, Arscott-Mills T, et al. Factors associated with parental readiness to make changes for overweight children. Pediatrics 2005;116(1): e94–101.
120. Berkowitz RI, Fujioka K, Daniels SR, et al. Effects of sibutramine treatment in obese adolescents: a randomized trial. Ann Intern Med 2006;145:81–90.
121. Berkowitz RI, Wadden TA, Tershakovec AM, et al. Behavior therapy and sibutramine for the treatment of adolescent obesity: a randomized controlled trial. JAMA 2003;289:1805–12.
122. Chanoine JP, Hampl S, Jensen C, et al. Effect of orlistat on weight and body composition in obese adolescents: a randomized controlled trial. JAMA 2005; 293:2873–83.
123. Bray GA. Medical therapy for obesity: current status and future hopes. Med Clin North Am 2007;91(6):1225–53.
124. Ortega-Gonzalez C, Luna S, Hernandez L, et al. Responses of serum androgen and insulin resistance to metformin and pioglitazone in obese, insulin-resistant women with polycystic ovary syndrome. J Clin Endocrinol Metab 2005;90(3): 1360–5.
125. Pittler MH, Ernst E. Dietary supplements for body-weight reduction: a systematic review. Am J Clin Nutr 2004;79(4):529–36.
126. Strauss RS, Bradley LJ, Brolin RE. Gastric bypass surgery in adolescents with morbid obesity. J Pediatr 2001;138:499–504.
127. Inge TH, Krebs NF, Garcia VF, et al. Bariatric surgery for severely overweight adolescents: concerns and recommendations. Pediatrics 2004;114:217–23.

Obesity in Pregnancy

Esa Davis, MD, MPH[a,*], Christine Olson, PhD[b]

KEYWORDS

- Pregnancy weight gain • Maternal obesity
- Postpartum weight retention • Gestational diabetes
- Gestational hypertension • Parity
- Perinatal weight interventions • Disparities

Obesity is a major public health problem that disproportionately affects childbearing women.[1–3] During the past several decades, women continue to have twice the obesity prevalence as that in men.[1] Currently, two-thirds of women are overweight, of which a third are obese.[1] The obesity prevalence among childbearing women aged 20 to 39 years increased from 9% in 1970 to 29% in 2004.[2] A similar increase in obesity prevalence occurred among adolescent women aged 12 to 19 years, which increased from 5% in 1970 to 16% in 2004.[3] Having 1 child doubles the 5- and 10-year incidence of obesity compared with that in women who have never given birth.[4,5] Maternal obesity predisposes a person to diabetes, hypertension, cardiovascular disease, cancer, and premature death.[6–9]

CHILDBEARING AND OBESITY RISK

Childbearing contributes to the long-term development of obesity in women. Prepregnancy, pregnancy, and postpartum periods are critical to the obesity problem. Although the relationship of pregnancy and maternal weight has been a focus of research during the past 20 years, the level of evidence in the field is still developing. Most studies have been cross-sectional or prospective, with few randomized controlled trials. The level of evidence differs greatly in definitions of outcomes, rigor of methods, sample size, and composition, and use of measured versus self-reported weights makes the findings difficult to summarize across studies. Additionally, many of the large epidemiologic studies are performed in other countries on homogenous populations, such as Sweden, which limits the generalizability to other more diverse populations such as the United States. Despite these limitations, maternal obesity is receiving greater attention as a major health problem for women and their infants.

Funding support: Robert Wood Johnson Harold Amos Faculty Award and University Hospital Case Medical Center Faculty Award.
[a] Department of Family Medicine, Case Western Reserve University, 11001 Cedar Avenue, Suite 306, Cleveland, OH 44106, USA
[b] Division of Nutritional Services, 376 MVR Hall, Cornell University, Ithaca, NY 14853, USA
* Corresponding author.
E-mail address: esa.davis@case.edu (E. Davis).

Prim Care Clin Office Pract 36 (2009) 341–356
doi:10.1016/j.pop.2009.01.005 **primarycare.theclinics.com**
0095-4543/09/$ – see front matter

FACTORS ASSOCIATED WITH MATERNAL WEIGHT GAIN

Maternal weight gain throughout the perinatal period has emerged as an area in which to understand obesity development in women. Perinatal factors such as prepregnancy weight, excessive pregnancy weight gain, postpartum weight retention, and high parity are potential risk factors for weight gain and obesity.[10–17]

Prepregnancy Weight

Prepregnancy weight is an important risk factor for both weight gained during pregnancy and weight retained after childbirth; women who are overweight at the beginning of pregnancy are significantly heavier after pregnancy.[18] The Institute of Medicine (IOM) 1990 pregnancy weight gain guidelines define prepregnancy weight by the following categories: underweight (body mass index [BMI] <19.8 kg/m^2), normal weight (BMI 19.8–26.0 kg/m^2), overweight (BMI >26.0–29.0 kg/m^2), and obese (BMI >29.0 kg/m^2); these differ from the World Health Organization guidelines.[19,20] Women who are obese prepregnancy are more likely than the normal prepregnancy weight women to have adverse pregnancy-related outcomes, such as gestational diabetes, pregnancy-induced hypertension, maternal infections, operative delivery, and neonatal hypoglycemia.[21]

Pregnancy Weight Gain

Physiologic changes

Total pregnancy weight gain, also known as maternal weight gain or gestational weight gain, comprises several components necessary to support the growth of the fetus and sustain the mother, which include maternal organs (uterus, breast, and blood), maternal adipose tissue reserves, and products of conception (placenta and fetus). Women double their blood volume, and the ligaments and joints relax to accommodate an expanding uterus. Mammary glands grow rapidly in preparation for milk production, and maternal fat reserves increase to provide enough energy substrates to support the mother and growing baby. Maternal fat reserves comprise 30% to 40% of the total maternal weight gain.[22–24] Few studies have examined the longitudinal changes in maternal body composition during the perinatal period.[25–27] Body composition during pregnancy has been difficult to study secondary to the safety and feasibility of instruments, such as total body potassium and hydrodensitometry. Skinfold thickness has been used to determine that maternal fat accumulates centrally rather than peripherally.[28] To date, most studies use BMI to estimate body fat in pregnant women because of its safety and easy determination in the clinical setting.

Recommended pregnancy weight gain

Historically, recommendations for appropriate pregnancy weight gain have varied substantially from restricting women's weight in the early 1900s to recommending weight gain by the late 1900s. The initial aim of restricting women's weight gain in pregnancy was to prevent macrosomia (large babies) and the associated delivery complications (eg, cesarean sections) as well as to reduce the incidence of preeclampsia.[29] The first published study by Prochownick in 1901 provided the evidence that restricting food intake in pregnancy reduced birth weights by approximately 400 to 500 gm. Epidemiologic studies during the late 1960s and 1970s revealed a link between maternal weight and fetal growth.[30–32] High infant mortality and morbidity rates were concerning and related to low infant birth weights (<2500 gm) and very low birth weights (<1500 gm). Thus, to reduce infant mortality by increasing maternal pregnancy weight, the IOM developed the 1990 pregnancy weight gain recommendations, which are the standard in clinical practice to this day.[19]

The IOM 1990 pregnancy weight gain recommendations are for women with a single fetus to promote optimal infant birth weights (**Table 1**). The IOM guidelines categorize women by their prepregnancy BMI and then recommend a range of total weight gain during pregnancy.[19] The ranges represent the 15th and 85th percentile weight gains in a nationally representative sample of births that produced a full-term baby of optimal birth size (3000 to 4000 g), which at the time had the lowest risk of mortality and morbidity. No defined upper limit of weight gain for obese women exists, and the recommendations are not applicable for women with multiple gestations. Recent research shows that the range of pregnancy weight gain recommended by the IOM continues to be associated with the optimal birth size of 3000 to 4000 gm, as originally defined.[33] Additionally, the IOM-recommended ranges are associated with decreased risk of bearing an infant with low birth weight (<2500 grams), macrosomia (>4000 g), small for gestational age, or large for gestational age (LGA). The relationship appears to be stronger in low- and normal-BMI women than that in the overweight- and obese-BMI women.[34] Due to this, the IOM is investigating these weight gain recommendations and the evidence behind them, but no changes are currently recommended.

Excess pregnancy weight gain

The increase in maternal obesity, particularly in the past decade since the guidelines were established, has raised concern whether they need to be revised. Approximately 30% to 40% of women are gaining weight within the recommended ranges.[13,35–37] Gaining weight more than the recommended IOM ranges has adverse effects for the mother and the baby, but why this happens is still being determined. Provider advice about recommended weight gain correlates strongly with actual pregnancy weight gain. Half of the women in a telephone survey reported receiving no advice or inappropriate advice about how much weight to gain. Additionally, women who did not receive advice had pregnancy weight gains that were either less than or more than the recommended guidelines.[36]

In another study of women who delivered a full-term infant and received benefits from the Women, Infants and Children Nutrition Education Program, 60% of those in the overweight prepregnancy BMI group gained greater weight than that in the IOM recommended guidelines compared with 25% of women in the underweight prepregnancy BMI group.[38] Other determinants associated with excessive pregnancy weight gain are increased caloric intake from prepregnancy to pregnancy and decreased physical activity during pregnancy.[13] Studies on other potential biologic determinants, such as genetic factors, hormone levels, and energy balance, are limited.[39–42]

Postpartum Weight Retention

The postpartum period is another time of considerable change in energy intake, expenditure, and weight. Most women will return to their prepregnancy weight by

Table 1
Institute of Medicine 1990 pregnancy weight gain guidelines

Prepregnancy BMI (kg/m^2)	Recommended Pregnancy Weight Gain
Underweight, <19.8	28–40 lb
Normal, 19.8–26.0	25–35 lb
Overweight, 26.1–29.0	15–25 lb
Obese, >29.0	At least 15 lb

1 year after childbirth; however, an increasing number of women are retaining weight after childbirth. Few women, 15% to 28%, will reach their prepregnancy weight by 6 weeks postpartum.[43–45] Postpartum weight retention is defined as the 6-week, 6-month, or 1-year postpartum weight minus the prepregnancy weight. Although the studies are few, the estimated average postpartum weight retention is 3.3 lb to 3.7 lb at 6 months to 1 year, with a range up to 20 lb.[46]

Weight retention after childbirth increases the risk of obesity.[5,11,12,15,46] Approximately 14% to 20% of women retain more than 5 kg (11 lb) long term.[47] Women who retain more than 6 lb at 6 months after childbirth have considerably more weight gain (18.3 lb vs 5.3 lb) during the subsequent 10 years.[16] Women unable to lose their pregnancy weight by 6 months are more likely to go into their second pregnancy heavier and are at greater risk for long-term weight gain.[12,16] In one of the largest samples of women (n = 7000), 73% of the women weighed more at the onset of the second pregnancy than they did before their first pregnancy; the average interpregnancy weight change being +3.4 kg (7.5 lb).[46] In spite of these studies, no current consensus for a universal definition of excessive postpartum weight retention exists.

Determinants for postpartum weight retention include excessive pregnancy weight gain, high prepregnancy weight, African American race, low socioeconomic status, and the extremes of maternal age (≤17 years and ≥35 years).[13,14,16,46,48–51] Generally, women who gain excessive amounts of weight during pregnancy retain more weight postpartum. By using the 1988 National Maternal and Infant Health Survey, Keppel and Taffel[50] determined that a greater proportion of women who gain weight more than the IOM weight gain guidelines retain more than 14 pounds at 10 to 14 months postpartum. Among women who gain weight within the IOM guidelines, 35% of African American women retain more than 14 lb postpartum compared with ~8% of Caucasian women.[50] These findings suggest that African American women who gain weight within and more than the IOM guidelines are at risk of significant weight retention after childbirth.

Parity and Weight

Parity is commonly defined in research studies as the number of live births. A woman is considered nulliparous (never given birth), primiparous (given birth to 1 child), or multiparous (given birth to 2 or more children). Some studies have shown that having 1 or more children can double the 5- and 10-year incidence of obesity, and women having 3 or more children are significantly more likely to be overweight or obese compared with nulliparous women.[5,52–56] On the other hand, a few studies report that primiparous women are more likely to have greater pregnancy weight gain and major long-term weight gain compared with that of multiparous women and nulliparous women.[5,11,19] Conversely, several studies report little or no relationship between parity and obesity.[15,55,57,58] The inconsistency in the findings of these studies may relate to differences in definitions of outcome, study designs, or confounding by baseline obesity. Thus, further studies are needed to clarify the relationship between parity and weight gain and determine whether this relationship differs across race, socioeconomic status, and age.

MATERNAL AND INFANT OUTCOMES RELATED TO MATERNAL OBESITY

Maternal obesity during pregnancy contributes to adverse maternal and infant outcomes, such as an increased risk of miscarriages, gestational diabetes, and pregnancy-induced hypertensive disorders, as well as long-term obesity and related comorbidities.[21,59–61] Maternal obesity increases the risk of operative deliveries (cesarean sections, forceps delivery, and vacuum extraction), premature delivery, anesthesia complications, wound infections, and deep venous thromboses.[21,59–62] Obese mothers are also more likely to have shorter durations of breastfeeding.[63,64]

Maternal obesity contributes to adverse infant outcomes, including macrosomia (infant birth weight >90th percentile or >4000 g); LGA; shoulder dystocia; and intrauterine, neonatal, or infant mortality.[61] For normal-weight women prepregnancy, the incidence of pregnancy and delivery complications reaches 30% to 40% for those who gain greater than 18 kg (~40 lb) and is lowest among those who gained weight within the IOM guidelines (11.5–16.0 kg).[65]

Gestational Diabetes

Gestational diabetes is characterized by insulin resistance and severe glucose intolerance (identified generally during the second trimester), which resolve after childbirth.[66] Gestational diabetes occurs in about 1% to 14% of pregnant women, depending on the population and diagnostic tests used, and increases the risk of developing type 2 diabetes mellitus long term.[67] Gestational diabetes is also related to adverse infant outcomes, such as macrosomia, LGA, neonatal trauma, neonatal hypoglycemia, and cesarean deliveries.[21,61,68] Additionally, infants of mothers with gestational diabetes are at risk of developing obesity, glucose intolerance, and diabetes during adolescence and adulthood.[69]

Independent of pregnancy weight gain, being overweight or obese prepregnancy is a strong risk factor for gestational diabetes; obese women are 6 times more likely to have it than normal prepregnancy weight women.[70,71] Excessive pregnancy weight gain has not been consistently established as a risk factor for gestational diabetes, though. Several US studies report a positive relationship between pregnancy weight gain and abnormal glucose tolerance.[71–74] Conversely, other studies have found higher risk of gestational diabetes among women with lower pregnancy weight gains,[65,75,76] although several studies identify no association between pregnancy weight gain and gestational diabetes.[70,77–79] Once again, the data are inconsistent in this specific area due to limitations in methods and criteria for diagnosis of gestational diabetes, but women who are overweight or obese prepregnancy are at a higher risk of developing gestational diabetes.

Pregnancy-Induced Hypertension/Pre-Eclampsia

Pregnancy-induced hypertension is hypertension that occurs during pregnancy and has 4 classifications: (1) chronic hypertension (blood pressure >140/90 before 20 weeks' gestation); (2) pre-eclampsia and eclampsia; (3) pre-eclampsia superimposed on chronic hypertension; and (4) gestational hypertension (hypertension alone, which is transient during pregnancy and postpartum).[80] Pregnancy-induced hypertension causes significant morbidity, such as placental abruption, stroke, intrauterine growth restriction, and death for mother and baby.[80,81] Pregnancy-induced hypertension increases the risk of developing essential hypertension long term.

Pre-eclampsia is characterized by hypertension (blood pressure >140/90), fluid retention (edema), and albuminuria, which develop after 20 weeks' gestation and generally reverses within 6 weeks after delivery. Pre-eclampsia complicates 3% to 5% of all pregnancies (10% of first-time pregnancies) and can progress to eclampsia, which is characterized by seizures.[80] The correlation between pregnancy weight gain and pre-eclampsia was one of the original reasons for restricting women's weight gain before the IOM guidelines. The rise in maternal obesity since the implementation of the IOM guidelines is concerning because of an increase in pregnancy-induced hypertension disorders.

The relationship of increasing pregnancy weight gain and pregnancy-induced hypertension has been fairly well established.[61] Pregnancy-induced hypertension disorders, in particular pre-eclampsia, occur most often in obese women.[70,82–84] Obese women with BMI greater than or equal to 29 prepregnancy are 2.2 times and 2.1 times more likely to develop gestational hypertension and pre-eclampsia, respectively, compared with normal-weight women.[85] The risk of pre-eclampsia increases with pregnancy weight gains greater than 25 lb among obese women.[86] For normal-weight women who gain weight more than the IOM guidelines (>35 lb), studies conflict—some state there is no association, whereas others note an association with greater risks of developing pre-eclampsia.[65] Another study showed that despite the prepregnancy BMI, those who gain more than 35 lb are at greater risk of developing pre-eclampsia.[87] More studies are necessary to determine a relationship between normal prepregnancy weight and pre-eclampsia, but a relationship is known between obese pregnant women and the development of pre-eclampsia.

Infant Outcomes

Despite the increase in birth weights and decrease in low birth weight and very low birth weight infants that have resulted from the implementation of the IOM 1990 guidelines, infant mortality rates have only modestly decreased. Women with weight gains more than the IOM guidelines or women overweight or obese entering pregnancy have greater adverse infant outcomes, such as head trauma, fractured clavicles, brachial plexus lesions, shoulder dystocia, increased risk of intrauterine fetal death, and infant mortality (death within the first year of life).[88] Obese women with a prepregnancy BMI greater than or equal to 30 have infant death risk during the perinatal period of 2.0 to 4.3 times that of normal prepregnancy weight mothers.[89,90]

Women who gain weight more than the IOM guidelines have twice the risk of having a macrosomic or LGA (>4500 g) infant and a 20% to 30% increase in having a cesarean delivery.[37] Compared with 4% of women with appropriate weight gain having LGA infants, 10% of normal prepregnant weight women who gain weight more than the IOM guidelines have LGA infants.[65]

SPECIAL HIGH-RISK POPULATIONS

Adolescents, women of low socioeconomic status, African American women, and women who have undergone bariatric surgery are at high risk for excessive gestational weight gain or postpartum weight retention. The common practice has been to recommend adolescents and African Americans to gain at the upper end of the pregnancy weight gain ranges to prevent low infant birth weights, which occur more frequently in these populations. More research is needed to characterize the pregnancy weight gain patterns of adolescents and determine whether the current adult guidelines need to be revised to accommodate the growing adolescent. African American and poor women have greater prepregnancy weight, parity, postpartum weight retention, and calorie intake, as well as decreased physical activity in the postpartum period.[11–13,16,17,46,48,51,91,92] African American women are twice as likely as Caucasian women to retain at least 20 lb postpartum.[46] High parity is also a risk factor for later-life obesity in African American women.[5,52] Interestingly, similar socioeconomic characteristics, such as low income and low educational level, are associated with gaining weight both more than and less than the IOM guidelines.[13]

Presently, minority, young, and primiparous women appear to be at increased risk of excessive gestational weight gain and postpartum weight retention, and there is a need for additional research on optimal pregnancy weight gains for these various groups. Additionally, not much is known about women who have undergone bariatric surgery and the appropriate pregnancy weight gains for this group. With the rise in bariatric procedures to reduce obesity becoming more prevalent, research is needed to understand the appropriate perinatal weight changes.

CURRENT CLINICAL PRACTICES AND INTERVENTIONS

To prevent maternal obesity, current weight loss interventions have primarily targeted excessive weight gain in pregnancy and postpartum weight retention. Developing and implementing effective weight loss interventions for peripartum women is challenging. To date, 5 clinical intervention studies have aimed to promote healthy weight gain during pregnancy.[93–97] All 5 studies contained an intervention to increase physical activity and promote healthy eating and behaviors (eg, goal setting and self-monitoring). The implementation of these 5 studies varied in intensity from mailing newsletters and health booklets to counseling sessions with dieticians, aqua aerobic classes, or weight monitoring by health providers. Most of these studies showed modest effectiveness in preventing excessive pregnancy weight gain.[93,95–97] The prevalence of excessive gestational weight gain in normal prepregnancy weight women can be decreased by about 40% with behavioral and educational intervention.[95,96]

Clinical interventions that focus on restricting maternal weight during pregnancy are controversial because of the strong association between maternal weight and infant birth weight. Thus, more research is needed to clarify the effects of limiting pregnancy weight gain on infant birth weight and outcomes. As of now, these limited studies provide evidence that monitoring weight gain during pregnancy, providing dietary and physical activity education and counseling, and providing materials that encourage behaviors, such as self-monitoring and goal setting, can promote healthy weight gain during pregnancy.

Weight loss interventions that reduce postpartum weight retention are a more recent effort to prevent maternal obesity. Four clinical intervention studies have focused on helping women return to their prepregnancy weight or less than their prepregnancy weight during the first year postpartum (**Table 2**).[98–101] These clinical intervention studies included diet, physical activity, and behavior modification delivered in a variety of ways, including educational group sessions, telephone contact, cooking sessions, and individual and group counseling sessions by trained nurses or paraprofessionals. Additionally, the intervention included components such as self-monitoring, keeping diet and physical activity diaries, goal setting, and written assignments on how to reduce calories and increase the consumption of fruit and vegetables, which the women were able to do at home.

All 4 studies had similar findings of more weight reduction postpartum in the treatment group compared with that in the control group. However, in 2 of the studies, there was minimal to no change in diet and physical activity behavior with weight loss between the treatment and control groups.[99,100] Self-monitoring appeared to be effective in helping women lose weight postpartum.

Although none of the interventions were delivered by physicians, physicians are essential to helping women manage their weight postpartum. Women's pregnancy weight gains tend to follow the recommendations of health care providers (eg, doctors, nurses, or nutrition counselors). Provider advice correlates significantly with the appropriate pregnancy weight gain range reported by women.[102] However, 18% of providers are giving women incorrect advice, and 33% are giving no advice regarding the appropriate weight gain in pregnancy.[36,102]

Table 2
Clinical intervention studies on reducing postpartum weight retention

Author (Reference)	Design	Study Population	Intervention	Weight Outcome
Leermakers et al[100]	Randomized controlled trial	97% White US ♀, age >18 y, 3–12 mo postpartum, exceed prepregnancy weight by 6.8 kg Control grp 43 Tx grp 47	Correspondence behavioral weight loss program for 6 mo- focused on low-fat/low-cal eating and increased physical activity: 2 grp sessions: self-monitoring techniques strategies to modify diet and exercise behavior correspondence materials telephone contact	33% of ♀ Tx grp vs 11.5% of control grp return to prepregnancy weight or less than prepregnancy weight Tx grp loss 7.8 kg vs 4.9 kg in control grp; $P<.03$ Tx grp loss 10.0 ± 5.8% pretreatment body weight vs 5.8 ± 5.7%, $P<.005$ Significant correlation with self-monitoring records and weight loss No relationship between phone contact or eating or exercising behavior and weight loss
Kinnunen et al[99]	Clinical trial	Primiparous Finnish ♀ age >18 y, normal and overweight, 2–10 mo postpartum Control grp 37 Tx grp 43	Dietary and physical activity counseling delivered by public health nurses during 5 clinic visits (2, 3, 5, 6, 10 mo)	50% Tx grp vs 30% control grp returned to their prepregnancy weight by 10 mo postpartum (not statistically significant) No between-grp differences found in intake of vegetables, fruit, or high-sugar snacks or leisure time physical activity

O'Toole et al[101]	Randomized controlled trial	99% White overweight US ♀, age >18 y, 6 wk–6 mo postpartum, gained 15 kg during pregnancy STR grp 21 SELF grp 19	STR:Individualized diet & exercise plans Food & activity diaries Grp educational sessions, vs self-directed intervention (SELF) Met for single 1-h educational session with dietician & exercise physiologist	STR grp mean weight loss 5.6 kg at 12 wk and 7.3 kg at 1 y postpartum Body weight unchanged for the SELF grp At 1 y postpartum, mean intakes were less than recommended for both grps: STR 309 kcal/d vs SELF 240 kcal/d Exercise was increased at 12 wk and 1 y postpartum for the STR grp and not SELF grp.
Bechtel-Blackwell[98]	Prospective, quasi-experimental	African American adolescent, primiparous♀, age 13–18 y receiving prenatal care Tx grp 22 Control grp 24	Nutrition education intervention Three 20-min grp sessions	Tx grp 11.9 lb retained less weight postpartum vs control grp 13.9 lb

Abbreviations: ♀, female; grp, group; SELF, self-directed intervention; STR, structured diet and physical activity intervention; Tx, treatment.

The postpartum period appears to be a good opportunity to address women's weight concerns and help them implement effective weight loss strategies. Conversely, the postpartum period is also a challenging time for new mothers attempting to balance their new roles and responsibilities. Competing demands for postpartum women hinder weight loss efforts and make participating in clinical trials challenging; this is evident in the small sample sizes and high attrition rates of the current intervention studies. Thus, effective weight loss interventions for women in the first year postpartum are still needed.

Until such studies are available, physicians and health care providers should monitor and counsel women on the appropriate weight gain prenatally. Ideally, encouraging overweight women to lose weight before pregnancy will help to prevent maternal obesity and associated adverse health outcomes for mother and baby. At the postpartum visit, women should discuss with their physician or health care provider plans for returning to their prepregnancy weight during the first year postpartum. The goal for weight loss for nonbreastfeeding, postpartum women is consistent with the current weight loss recommendations for nonpregnant women, which is 1 to 2 lb/wk. According to the IOM 1990 recommendations, a weight loss of ~0.5 to 1 lb/wk appears to be safe for overweight, lactating mothers.[103] Additionally, aerobic exercise without dietary restriction does not appear to reduce the volume of breast milk or affect composition.[104–106] Currently, there are no recommendations for dietary restriction for weight loss during lactation, because experimental studies have been few and inconclusive.[107–109] Thus, more studies are needed to determine whether dietary restriction during lactation is a safe and effective strategy for weight loss.

Comprehensive interventions may be difficult to implement in a busy clinical practice; however, health care providers can, at a minimum, help link women to resources in the community that may help them achieve their weight management goal. Additionally, patient education and counseling in nutrition and physical activity can be delivered by trained professionals, such as nurses and lay community workers, or delivered to women in less personnel-intensive ways, such as by mail, using well-designed self-help materials.

SUMMARY

Women of childbearing age have increasing rates of obesity. Having high prepregnancy weight, excessive pregnancy weight gain, and postpartum weight retention increases a woman's risk of weight gain and obesity long term. The IOM 1990 pregnancy weight gain guidelines are still the standard of care for optimizing infant birth weights, although the reasons for women gaining weight more than the recommendations still need to be determined.

Maternal obesity contributes to maternal and infant morbidity and mortality. Special populations, such as adolescents, African Americans, and women with low socioeconomic status, are at high risk for maternal obesity. Educating pregnant patients about appropriate weight gain, nutrition, and exercise is necessary in the clinical setting.

REFERENCES

1. Flegal KM, Carroll MD, Ogden CL, et al. Prevalence and trends in obesity among US adults, 1999–2000. JAMA 2002;288(14):1723–7.
2. Ogden CL, Carroll MD, Curtin LR, et al. Prevalence of overweight and obesity in the United States, 1999–2004. JAMA 2006;295(13):1549–55.

3. Ogden CL, Flegal KM, Carroll MD, et al. Prevalence and trends in overweight among US children and adolescents, 1999–2000. JAMA 2002;288(14): 1728–32.
4. Davis EM, Zyzanski SJ, Olson CM, et al. Racial, ethnic, and socioeconomic differences in the incidence of obesity related to childbirth. Am J Public Health 2009;99:294–9.
5. Williamson DF, Madans J, Pamuk E, et al. A prospective study of childbearing and 10-year weight gain in US white women 25 to 45 years of age. Int J Obes Relat Metab Disord 1994;18(8):561–9.
6. Brancati FL, Kao WH, Folsom AR, et al. Incident type 2 diabetes mellitus in African American and white adults: the Atherosclerosis Risk in Communities Study. JAMA 2000;283(17):2253–9.
7. Flegal KM, Graubard BI, Williamson DF. Methods of calculating deaths attributable to obesity. Am J Epidemiol 2004;160(4):331–8.
8. Flegal KM, Williamson DF, Graubard BI. Obesity and cancer. N Engl J Med 2003; 349(5):502–4.
9. Mokdad AH, Ford ES, Bowman BA, et al. Prevalence of obesity, diabetes, and obesity-related health risk factors, 2001. JAMA 2003;289(1):76–9.
10. Abrams B. Prenatal weight gain and postpartum weight retention: a delicate balance. Am J Public Health 1993;83(8):1082–4.
11. Harris HE, Ellison GT, Holliday M, et al. The impact of pregnancy on the long-term weight gain of primiparous women in England. Int J Obes Relat Metab Disord 1997;21(9):747–55.
12. Linne Y, Barkeling B, Rossner S. Long-term weight development after pregnancy. Obes Rev 2002;3(2):75–83.
13. Olson CM, Strawderman MS, Hinton PS, et al. Gestational weight gain and postpartum behaviors associated with weight change from early pregnancy to 1 y postpartum. Int J Obes Relat Metab Disord 2003;27(1):117–27.
14. Parham ES, Astrom MF, King SH. The association of pregnancy weight gain with the mother's postpartum weight. J Am Diet Assoc 1990;90(4):550–4.
15. Rookus MA, Rokebrand P, Burema J, et al. The effect of pregnancy on the body mass index 9 months postpartum in 49 women. Int J Obes 1987;11(6): 609–18.
16. Rooney BL, Schauberger CW. Excess pregnancy weight gain and long-term obesity: one decade later. Obstet Gynecol 2002;100(2):245–52.
17. Wolfe WS, Sobal J, Olson CM, et al. Parity-associated weight gain and its modification by sociodemographic and behavioral factors: a prospective analysis in US women. Int J Obes Relat Metab Disord 1997;21(9):802–10.
18. McKeown T, Record R. The Influence of weight and height on weight changes associated with pregnancy in women. J Endocrinol 1957;15:423–9.
19. Institute of Medicine. Nutrition during pregnancy. Washington, DC: National Academy Press; 1990.
20. WHO. Obesity: preventing and managing the global Epidemic. Report of a WHO Consultation of Obesity. Geneva 1997. June 3–5.
21. Doherty DA, Magann EF, Francis J, et al. Pre-pregnancy body mass index and pregnancy outcomes. Int J Gynaecol Obstet 2006;95(3):242–7.
22. Butte NF, Ellis KJ, Wong WW, et al. Composition of gestational weight gain impacts maternal fat retention and infant birth weight. Am J Obstet Gynecol 2003;189(5):1423–32.
23. Durnin JV. Energy requirements of pregnancy. Acta Paediatr Scand Suppl 1991; 373:33–42.

24. Kopp-Hoolihan LE, van Loan MD, Wong WW, et al. Fat mass deposition during pregnancy using a four-component model. J Appl Phys 1999;87(1):196–202.
25. Forsum E, Sadurskis A, Wager J. Estimation of body fat in healthy Swedish women during pregnancy and lactation. Am J Clin Nutr 1989;50(3):465–73.
26. Lederman SA, Pierson RN Jr, Wang J, et al. Body composition measurements during pregnancy. Basic Life Sci 1993;60:193–5.
27. Lindsay CA, Huston L, Amini SB, et al. Longitudinal changes in the relationship between body mass index and percent body fat in pregnancy. Obstet Gynecol 1997;89(3):377–82.
28. Taggart NR, Holliday RM, Billewicz WZ, et al. Changes in skinfolds during pregnancy. Br J Nutr 1967;21(2):439–51.
29. McIlroy A, Rodway H. Weight-changes during and after pregnancy with special reference to early diagnosis of toxaemia. J Obstet Gynaecol 1937;44:221–44.
30. Billewicz WC, Thomson AM. Clinical significance of weight trends during pregnancy. Br Med J 1957;1(5013):243–7.
31. Eastman NJ, Jackson E. Weight relationships in pregnancy. I. The bearing of maternal weight gain and pre-pregnancy weight on birth weight in full term pregnancies. Obstet Gynecol Surv 1968;23(11):1003–25.
32. Singer JE, Westphal M, Niswander K. Relationship of weight gain during pregnancy to birth weight and infant growth and development in the first year of life. Obstet Gynecol 1968;31(3):417–23.
33. Lederman SA. Pregnancy weight gain and postpartum loss: avoiding obesity while optimizing the growth and development of the fetus. J Am Med Womens Assoc 2001;56(2):53–8.
34. Olson CM. Achieving a healthy weight gain during pregnancy. Annu Rev Nutr 2008;28:411–23.
35. Caulfield LE, Witter FR, Stoltzfus RJ. Determinants of gestational weight gain outside the recommended ranges among black and white women. Obstet Gynecol 1996;87(5 Pt 1):760–6.
36. Cogswell ME, Scanlon KS, Fein SB, et al. Medically advised, mother's personal target, and actual weight gain during pregnancy. Obstet Gynecol 1999;94(4):616–22.
37. Parker JD, Abrams B. Prenatal weight gain advice: an examination of the recent prenatal weight gain recommendations of the Institute of Medicine. Obstet Gynecol 1992;79(5 Pt 1):664–9.
38. Schieve LA, Cogswell ME, Scanlon KS. Trends in pregnancy weight gain within and outside ranges recommended by the Institute of Medicine in a WIC population. Matern Child Health J 1998;2(2):111–6.
39. Dishy V, Gupta S, Landau R, et al. G-protein beta(3) subunit 825 C/T polymorphism is associated with weight gain during pregnancy. Pharmacogenetics 2003;13(4):241–2.
40. Scholl TO, Chen X. Insulin and the "thrifty" woman: the influence of insulin during pregnancy on gestational weight gain and postpartum weight retention. Matern Child Health J 2002;6(4):255–61.
41. Stein TP, Scholl TO, Schluter MD, et al. Plasma leptin influences gestational weight gain and postpartum weight retention. Am J Clin Nutr 1998;68(6):1236–40.
42. Tok EC, Ertunc D, Bilgin O, et al. PPAR-gamma2 Pro12Ala polymorphism is associated with weight gain in women with gestational diabetes mellitus. Eur J Obstet Gynecol Reprod Biol 2006;129(1):25–30.
43. Olsen LC, Mundt MH. Postpartum weight loss in a nurse-midwifery practice. J Nurse Midwifery 1986;31(4):177–81.

44. Schauberger CW, Rooney BL, Brimer LM. Factors that influence weight loss in the puerperium. Obstet Gynecol 1992;79(3):424–9.
45. Walker LO, Timmerman GM, Sterling BS, et al. Do low-income women attain their pre-pregnant weight by the 6th week of postpartum? Ethn Dis 2004;14(1):119–26.
46. Greene GW, Smiciklas-Wright H, Scholl TO, et al. Postpartum weight change: how much of the weight gained in pregnancy will be lost after delivery? Obstet Gynecol 1988;71(5):701–7.
47. Gunderson EP, Abrams B. Epidemiology of gestational weight gain and body weight changes after pregnancy. Epidemiol Rev 1999;21(2):261–75.
48. Boardley DJ, Sargent RG, Coker AL, et al. The relationship between diet, activity, and other factors, and postpartum weight change by race. Obstet Gynecol 1995;86(5):834–8.
49. Gunderson EP, Abrams B, Selvin S. Does the pattern of postpartum weight change differ according to pregravid body size? Int J Obes Relat Metab Disord 2001;25(6):853–62.
50. Keppel KG, Taffel SM. Pregnancy-related weight gain and retention: implications of the 1990 Institute of Medicine guidelines. Am J Public Health 1993;83(8): 1100–3.
51. Parker JD, Abrams B. Differences in postpartum weight retention between black and white mothers. Obstet Gynecol 1993;81(5 Pt 1):768–74.
52. Burke GL, Savage PJ, Manolio TA, et al. Correlates of obesity in young black and white women: the CARDIA Study. Am J Public Health 1992;82(12):1621–5.
53. Arroyo P, Avila-Rosas H, Fernandez V, et al. Parity and the prevalence of overweight. Int J Gynaecol Obstet 1995;48(3):269–72.
54. Billewicz WZ. Body weight in parous women. Br J Prev Soc Med 1970;24(2): 97–104.
55. Brown JE, Kaye SA, Folsom AR. Parity-related weight change in women. Int J Obes Relat Metab Disord 1992;16(9):627–31.
56. Heliovaara M, Aromaa A. Parity and obesity. J Epidemiol Community Health 1981;35(3):197–9.
57. Lee SK, Sobal J, Frongillo EA, et al. Parity and body weight in the United States: differences by race and size of place of residence. Obes Res 2005;13(7): 1263–9.
58. Coitinho DC, Sichieri R, D'Aquino Benicio MH. Obesity and weight change related to parity and breast-feeding among parous women in Brazil. Public Health Nutr 2001;4(4):865–70.
59. Barau G, Robillard PY, Hulsey TC, et al. Linear association between maternal pre-pregnancy body mass index and risk of caesarean section in term deliveries. BJOG 2006;113(10):1173–7.
60. Robinson HE, O'Connell CM, Joseph KS, et al. Maternal outcomes in pregnancies complicated by obesity. Obstet Gynecol 2005;106(6):1357–64.
61. Viswanathan M, Siega-Riz AM, Moos MK, et al. Outcomes of maternal weight gain, Evidence Report/Technology Assessment No. 168. Rockville (MD): Agency for Healthcare Research and Quality; 2008.
62. Dietz PM, Callaghan WM, Morrow B, et al. Population-based assessment of the risk of primary cesarean delivery due to excess prepregnancy weight among nulliparous women delivering term infants. Matern Child Health J 2005;9(3): 237–44.
63. Hilson JA, Rasmussen KM, Kjolhede CL. Excessive weight gain during pregnancy is associated with earlier termination of breast-feeding among White women. J Nutr 2006;136(1):140–6.

64. Hilson JA, Rasmussen KM, Kjolhede CL. High prepregnant body mass index is associated with poor lactation outcomes among white, rural women independent of psychosocial and demographic correlates. J Hum Lact 2004;20(1):18–29.
65. Thorsdottir I, Torfadottir JE, Birgisdottir BE, et al. Weight gain in women of normal weight before pregnancy: complications in pregnancy or delivery and birth outcome. Obstet Gynecol 2002;99(5 Pt 1):799–806.
66. Catalano PM, Kirwan JP, Haugel-de Mouzon S, et al. Gestational diabetes and insulin resistance: role in short- and long-term implications for mother and fetus. J Nutr 2003;133(5 Suppl 2):1674S–83S.
67. Damm P. Gestational diabetes mellitus and subsequent development of overt diabetes mellitus. Dan Med Bull 1998;45(5):495–509.
68. Hod M, Merlob P, Friedman S, et al. Prevalence of minor congenital anomalies in newborns of diabetic mothers. Eur J Obstet Gynecol Reprod Biol 1992;44(2): 111–6.
69. Metzger BE, Coustan DR. Summary and recommendations of the Fourth International Workshop-Conference on Gestational Diabetes Mellitus. The Organizing Committee. Diabetes Care 1998;21(Suppl 2):B161–7.
70. Bianco AT, Smilen SW, Davis Y, et al. Pregnancy outcome and weight gain recommendations for the morbidly obese woman. Obstet Gynecol 1998;91(1): 97–102.
71. Saldana TM, Siega-Riz AM, Adair LS, et al. The relationship between pregnancy weight gain and glucose tolerance status among black and white women in central North Carolina. Am J Obstet Gynecol 2006;195(6):1629–35.
72. Edwards LE, Hellerstedt WL, Alton IR, et al. Pregnancy complications and birth outcomes in obese and normal-weight women: effects of gestational weight change. Obstet Gynecol 1996;87(3):389–94.
73. Kabiru W, Raynor BD. Obstetric outcomes associated with increase in BMI category during pregnancy. Am J Obstet Gynecol 2004;191(3):928–32.
74. Kieffer EC, Carman WJ, Gillespie BW, et al. Obesity and gestational diabetes among African-American women and Latinas in Detroit: implications for disparities in women's health. J Am Med Womens Assoc 2001;56(4):181–7, 196.
75. Brennand EA, Dannenbaum D, Willows ND. Pregnancy outcomes of First Nations women in relation to pregravid weight and pregnancy weight gain. J Obstet Gynaecol Can 2005;27(10):936–44.
76. Kieffer EC, Tabaei BP, Carman WJ, et al. The influence of maternal weight and glucose tolerance on infant birthweight in Latino mother-infant pairs. Am J Public Health 2006;96(12):2201–8.
77. Hackmon R, James R, O'Reilly Green C, et al. The impact of maternal age, body mass index and maternal weight gain on the glucose challenge test in pregnancy. J Matern Fetal Neonatal Med 2007;20(3):253–7.
78. Murakami M, Ohmichi M, Takahashi T, et al. Prepregnancy body mass index as an important predictor of perinatal outcomes in Japanese. Arch Gynecol Obstet 2005;271(4):311–5.
79. Seghieri G, De Bellis A, Anichini R, et al. Does parity increase insulin resistance during pregnancy? Diabet Med 2005;22(11):1574–80.
80. Report of the National High Blood Pressure Education Program Working Group on High Blood Pressure in Pregnancy. Am J Obstet Gynecol 2000;183(1):S1–22.
81. Rochat RW, Koonin LM, Atrash HK, et al. Maternal mortality in the United States: report from the Maternal Mortality Collaborative. Obstet Gynecol 1988;72(1): 91–7.

82. Jensen DM, Ovesen P, Beck-Nielsen H, et al. Gestational weight gain and pregnancy outcomes in 481 obese glucose-tolerant women. Diabetes Care 2005; 28(9):2118–22.
83. Keil JE, Gazes PC, Sutherland SE, et al. Predictors of physical disability in elderly blacks and whites of the Charleston Heart Study. J Clin Epidemiol 1989;42(6):521–9.
84. Sibai BM, Gordon T, Thom E, et al. Risk factors for preeclampsia in healthy nulliparous women: a prospective multicenter study. The National Institute of Child Health and Human Development Network of Maternal-Fetal Medicine Units. Am J Obstet Gynecol 1995;172(2 Pt 1):642–8.
85. Thadhani R, Stampfer MJ, Hunter DJ, et al. High body mass index and hypercholesterolemia: risk of hypertensive disorders of pregnancy. Obstet Gynecol 1999;94(4):543–50.
86. Kiel DW, Dodson EA, Artal R, et al. Gestational weight gain and pregnancy outcomes in obese women: how much is enough? Obstet Gynecol 2007; 110(4):752–8.
87. Cedergren M. Effects of gestational weight gain and body mass index on obstetric outcome in Sweden. Int J Gynaecol Obstet 2006;93(3):269–74.
88. Baeten JM, Bukusi EA, Lambe M. Pregnancy complications and outcomes among overweight and obese nulliparous women. Am J Public Health 2001; 91(3):436–40.
89. Cnattingius S, Bergstrom R, Lipworth L, et al. Prepregnancy weight and the risk of adverse pregnancy outcomes. N Engl J Med 1998;338(3):147–52.
90. Naeye RL. Maternal body weight and pregnancy outcome. Am J Clin Nutr 1990; 52(2):273–9.
91. Howie LD, Parker JD, Schoendorf KC. Excessive maternal weight gain patterns in adolescents. J Am Diet Assoc 2003;103(12):1653–7.
92. Rosenberg L, Palmer JR, Adams-Campbell LL, et al. Obesity and hypertension among college-educated black women in the United States. J Hum Hypertens 1999;13(4):237–41.
93. Claesson IM, Sydsjo G, Brynhildsen J, et al. Weight gain restriction for obese pregnant women: a case-control intervention study. BJOG 2008;115(1):44–50.
94. Kinnunen TI, Pasanen M, Aittasalo M, et al. Preventing excessive weight gain during pregnancy - a controlled trial in primary health care. Eur J Clin Nutr 2007;61(7):884–91.
95. Olson CM, Strawderman MS, Reed RG. Efficacy of an intervention to prevent excessive gestational weight gain. Am J Obstet Gynecol 2004;191(2):530–6.
96. Polley BA, Wing RR, Sims CJ. Randomized controlled trial to prevent excessive weight gain in pregnant women. Int J Obes Relat Metab Disord 2002;26(11): 1494–502.
97. Wolff S, Legarth J, Vangsgaard K, et al. A randomized trial of the effects of dietary counseling on gestational weight gain and glucose metabolism in obese pregnant women. Int J Obes (Lond) 2008;32(3):495–501.
98. Bechtel-Blackwell DA. Computer-assisted self-interview and nutrition education in pregnant teens. Clin Nurs Res 2002;11(4):450–62.
99. Kinnunen TI, Pasanen M, Aittasalo M, et al. Reducing postpartum weight retention–a pilot trial in primary health care. Nutr J 2007;6:21.
100. Leermakers EA, Anglin K, Wing RR. Reducing postpartum weight retention through a correspondence intervention. Int J Obes Relat Metab Disord 1998; 22(11):1103–9.

101. O'Toole ML, Sawicki MA, Artal R. Structured diet and physical activity prevent postpartum weight retention. J Womens Health (Larchmt) 2003;12(10):991–8.
102. Stotland NE, Haas JS, Brawarsky P, et al. Body mass index, provider advice, and target gestational weight gain. Obstet Gynecol 2005;105(3):633–8.
103. Institute of Medicine. Nutrition during lactation. Washington, DC: National Academy Press; 1991.
104. Dewey KG, Lovelady CA, Nommsen-Rivers LA, et al. A randomized study of the effects of aerobic exercise by lactating women on breast-milk volume and composition. N Engl J Med 1994;330(7):449–53.
105. Lovelady CA, Lonnerdal B, Dewey KG. Lactation performance of exercising women. Am J Clin Nutr 1990;52(1):103–9.
106. Lovelady CA, Nommsen-Rivers LA, McCrory MA, et al. Effects of exercise on plasma lipids and metabolism of lactating women. Med Sci Sports Exerc 1995;27(1):22–8.
107. Dusdieker LB, Hemingway DL, Stumbo PJ. Is milk production impaired by dieting during lactation? Am J Clin Nutr 1994;59(4):833–40.
108. McCrory MA, Nommsen-Rivers LA, Mole PA, et al. Randomized trial of the short-term effects of dieting compared with dieting plus aerobic exercise on lactation performance. Am J Clin Nutr 1999;69(5):959–67.
109. Strode MA, Dewey KG, Lonnerdal B. Effects of short-term caloric restriction on lactational performance of well-nourished women. Acta Paediatr Scand 1986; 75(2):222–9.

Nutritional Treatment of Obesity

Roger A. Shewmake, PhD, LN[a,b,*], Mark K. Huntington, MD, PhD, FAAFP[a,b]

KEYWORDS

- Nutrition • Weight loss • Supplements
- Diet • Low-fat • Low-carb

PRINCIPLES OF NUTRITION

Dietary Guidelines for Americans

The Food and Nutrition Board of the Institute of Medicine (IOM) along with Health Canada have released the sixth in a series of reports on dietary reference values for the intake of macronutrients and energy for Americans and Canadians.[1] The guidelines set Dietary Reference Intakes (DRIs) for carbohydrates, fiber, fatty acids, cholesterol, protein, amino acids, energy, and physical activity. The new DRIs replace the older recommended dietary allowances last updated in 1989. The DRIs are based on evidence of relationships between nutrient intake and prevention of chronic disease as well as the maintenance of good health.

Two major goals are set forth in the new dietary guidelines: (1) create a message that will inspire individuals to look for more information about healthy eating; and (2) communicate scientifically accurate concepts that are understandable and meaningful. Confusion from marketing and food label terminology, such as "whole grain," "organic," "fat-free," "no trans fats," "all natural," "rich in fiber," "low glycemic index (GI)," "lowers cholesterol," and so on, occurs. Forty-one key recommendations are identified in the guidelines, 23 for the general public and 18 for special populations. Nine general topics, including adequate nutrients within calorie needs, weight management, physical activity, food groups to encourage, fats, carbohydrates, sodium, and potassium, alcoholic beverages, and food safety, are covered. Health education experts are provided with a compilation of the latest evidence-based nutrition and physical activity recommendations. The guidelines are also used as a basis of federal nutrition policy and education and are also designed to help the public make healthier choices about food and physical activity.

[a] Department of Family Medicine, Sanford School of Medicine, University of South Dakota, 1400 West 22nd Street, Sioux Falls, SD 57105, USA

[b] Sioux Falls Family Medicine Residency Program, Center for Family Medicine, 1115 East 20th Street, Sioux Falls, SD 57110, USA

* Corresponding author. Sioux Falls Family Medicine Residency Program, Center for Family Medicine, 1115 East 20th Street, Sioux Falls, SD 57110.

E-mail address: roger.shewmake@usd.edu (R.A. Shewmake).

Prim Care Clin Office Pract 36 (2009) 357–377
doi:10.1016/j.pop.2009.01.010 primarycare.theclinics.com
0095-4543/09/$ – see front matter

The guidelines provide evidence-based advice for ages 2 plus in an effort to promote health and prevent chronic disease. They also help guide federal policy and programs. Various implementation tools are provided by the guidelines, including the Dietary Approaches to Stop Hypertension (DASH) eating plan,[2] interpreting the food label, the US Food Guidance System (FGS), and Toolkit for Nutritional Professionals.

The guidelines emphasize consuming a variety of nutrient-dense foods and beverages from the basic food groups. Choices should limit intake of saturated and trans fat, cholesterol, added sugars, salt, and alcohol. The DASH diet and the FGS are provided as examples of healthy eating patterns. Food groups identified with disease prevention are delineated, and specific recommendations are made for people over 50 years, women who may become pregnant and those in the first trimester, older adults, dark-skinned people, and people exposed to insufficient ultraviolet B radiation.

FOOD GROUPS TO ENCOURAGE

Carbohydrates

Selection of fiber-rich fruits, vegetables, and whole grains is recommended. Choosing and preparing foods and beverages with little added sugar or caloric sweetener, such as amounts suggested by the DASH eating plan and FGS, are also recommended. The new guidelines have a focus on fiber that had not occurred in previous editions. Specific recommendations for children and adolescents include the suggestion that at least half the grains should be from whole-grain sources.

Fats

Sources of fat may also contribute potentially harmful cholesterol and saturated and trans fats. Metabolism of fats requires approximately 3% of dietary fat for conversion to body fat, whereas approximately 33% of dietary carbohydrate and protein is required for carbohydrate and protein conversion, respectively.[3]

Recommendations for consumption of saturated fats should be at less than 10% of calories and less than 300 mg/d of cholesterol, and trans-fatty acid consumption should be as low as possible. Total fat intake is recommended to be between 20% to 30%, with most fats coming from polyunsaturated fatty acids (PUFAs) and monounsaturated fatty acids (MUFAs), such as fish, nuts, and vegetable oils. Meats, poultry, dried beans, milk, or milk products that are low fat or fat free should be selected, with a limited intake of fats and oils high in saturated or trans-fatty acids. Total fat recommendations for children are 20% to 30% of total caloric intake and adolescents, for 2- to 3-year-olds, 30% to 35% of total caloric intake, and for those 4 to 8 years, 25% to 30% of total caloric intake, with most fats coming from PUFAs and MUFAs, such as fish, nuts, and vegetable oils.

Fiber

The indigestible component of plant foods is known as dietary fiber. There are 2 main types, soluble and insoluble. Each type has an important health benefit. Recommendations for fiber intake are presented in **Table 1**. Individuals over the age of 4 should be getting at least 25 g fiber each day, yet most do not get one-half of the recommendation.[4]

Insoluble fiber is an important aid in normal bowel function, promoting regularity and normalizing the gut. Foods high in insoluble fiber include the following: whole wheat breads, wheat cereals, wheat bran, rye, rice, barley, cabbage, beets, carrots, brussels sprouts, turnips, cauliflower, and apple skins.

Table 1
Fiber recommendations by age and gender

How Much Fiber Do I Need		
Children		
1–3 y	Boys & girls	19 g/d
4–8 y	Boys & girls	25 g/d
9–13 y	Boys Girls	31 g/d 26 g/d
14–18 y	Boys Girls	38 g/d 26 g/d
Adults		
19–50 y	Men Women	38 g/d 25 g/d
>50 y	Men Women	30 g/d 21 g/d

Data from Panel on Macronutrients, Panel on the Definition of Dietary Fiber, Subcommittee on Upper Reference Levels of Nutrients, et al. Dietary reference intakes for energy, carbohydrate, fiber, fat, fatty acids, cholesterol, protein, and amino acids (macronutrients). Washington, DC: National Academies Press; 2005.

Soluble fiber forms a gel that delays gastric emptying; therefore, carbohydrates from food do not enter the blood stream as rapidly and thus can minimize a sudden rise in blood glucose. Dietary soluble fiber also helps reduce the absorption of fat and cholesterol and interrupts enterohepatic circulation, thus decreasing its efficiency. Soluble fiber sources include oat bran, oatmeal, beans, peas, rice bran, barley, citrus fruits, apple pulp, psyllium, carrots, strawberries, peaches with skin, and apples with the skin.

Most fiber-rich foods often contain a mixture of both soluble and insoluble fibers. Eating a variety of high-fiber foods is recommended. Fiber, especially insoluble fiber, helps promote regularity. Individuals should gradually increase their dietary fiber intake over time and increase intake of fluids. Foods high in fiber tend to be lower in total calories, saturated fat, and cholesterol. A feeling of fullness and lessened appetite and/or hunger often result with increased consumption of fiber and can be an important adjunct to weight management plans.

Calcium

Many population groups do not meet National Academy of Sciences (NAS) daily calcium recommendations.[5] Seventy percent of preteen girls and 60% of preteen boys aged 6 to 11 years and nearly 90% of teen-aged girls and almost 70% of teen-aged boys in the age group of 12 to 19 years fall short of meeting their calcium needs. Low calcium intake is related to the increased risk of bone fractures in childhood, adolescents, and osteoporosis in adults. The American Academy of Pediatrics[6] issued a policy statement urging pediatricians to recommend milk, cheese, yogurt, and other calcium-rich foods for children's daily diets to help build their bone mass and prevent rickets. Children of 2 to 8 years should consume 2 cups of fat-free or low-fat milk or equivalent milk products per day.

Seventy-two percent of the calcium available in the US food supply comes from dairy products.[5] An 8-oz serving of milk provides about 35% of the 800-mg calcium recommended for children aged 4 through 8 years, 23% of the 1300 mg recommended for individuals aged 9 through 18 years, 30% of the 1000 mg recommended for adults 19 to 50 years of age, and 25% of the 1200 mg recommended for adults aged 51 years or older. The perception that dairy products and milk have a higher caloric content and, therefore, should be avoided to "lose weight" is an important contributing factor to reduced calcium intake.

The highest demand for calcium is among children and adolescents during rapid skeletal growth and among women during pregnancy and breastfeeding. Postmenopausal women and older men also need to consume more calcium. Low-fat dairy products, such as milk, yogurt, cheese, and ice cream, dark leafy green vegetables, such as spinach, broccoli, and various greens, bok choy, tofu, almonds, and fish, such as sardines and salmon with the bones, are good sources of calcium. Calcium-fortified foods include orange juice, breakfast cereals, and breads. The new calcium guidelines from the NAS[5] and the calcium content of selected foods are illustrated in **Tables 2** and **3**.

Sodium and Potassium

Consumption of 2300 mg of sodium (approximately 1 teaspoon of salt) or less per day is recommended for healthy individuals.[1] The American Heart Association recommends less than 1500 mg daily for those with hypertension.[7] Healthy adults between 19 and 50 years should consume about 4700 mg of potassium per day. A combination of choosing and preparing foods with little salt and at the same time consuming potassium-rich foods, such as fruits and vegetables, will help accomplish this goal. The potassium content of modern diets is low largely due to modern processing and high levels of salt added to most processed foods. In the past, potassium was more plentiful in the diet than salt, but gradually, the situation has been reversed. Potassium is abundant in fruits, vegetables, and dairy products (**Table 4**).

Alcoholic Beverages

For those who choose to drink alcoholic beverages, the US Dietary Guidelines 2005 recommend to do so sensibly and in moderation. Moderation is defined as the consumption of up to 1 drink per day for women and up to 2 drinks per day for men. A standard drink is considered to be 12 oz of beer, 1.5 oz of distilled spirit, or 5 oz of wine. Alcohol should not be consumed by some individuals and should be avoided by individuals engaging in activities that require attention, skill, or coordination. There is a dose-response relationship between alcohol and blood pressure

Table 2
Calcium recommendations

Calcium Guidelines	
Life Stage Group (y)	**Calcium Goal (mg/d)**
1–3	500
4–8	800
9–18	1300
19–50	1000
51+	1200
Pregnant or lactating	
≤18	1300
19–50	1000

Data from Standing Committee on the Scientific Evaluation of Dietary Reference Intakes FaNB, Institute of Medicine. Dietary reference intakes for calcium, phosphorus, magnesium, vitamin D, and fluoride. Washington, DC: National Academy Press; 1997.

Table 3
Calcium sources

Calcium Content of Selected Foods

Source	Calcium Content	Percent of DRI
Yogurt (1%, 1C)	452 mg	45
Sardines (8 medium)	354	35.4
Milk (1%, 1C)	300	30
Swiss cheese (1 oz)	259	32
Broccoli (1 stalk)	103	10.3
Spinach (3.5 oz, raw)	93	9.3
Shrimp (fried, 3.5 oz)	72	7.2

Abbreviation: C, cup.

(BP), especially in people drinking more than 2 drinks daily. Meta-analysis has shown that consuming less alcohol reduces both systolic and diastolic BP, and decreasing alcohol intake may lower BP by an average of 2 to 4 mm of mercury.

FOOD LABELS, CALORIES, AND NUTRIENT RECOMMENDATIONS

A new general guide to calories has been provided by the US Dietary Guidelines to aid consumers. Food labels indicate that 40 calories is considered a *low* consumption, 100 calories is *moderate*, and 400 calories is *high*, based on a 2000-calorie diet. The new food label recommendations offer consumers advice on which nutrients to increase and those to limit. The label is also helpful in indicating whether or not a product is a good source of nutrients.

LIFESTYLE INSTRUCTION AND BEHAVIORAL MODIFICATION

Successful weight control and healthy eating are based on behavioral changes that can be maintained for life. Helping patients to identify the needed changes in their

Table 4
Dietary sources of potassium

		Percent Minimum Requirement	
Source	**Potassium Content**	**2000 mg**	**3500 mg**
Molasses (2 T)	1500 mg	75%	43%
Beans (kidney, 1/2 C)	984 mg	49%	28%
Beans (pinto, 1/2 C)	984 mg	49%	28%
Raisins (1/2 C)	610 mg	31%	17%
Potato (without skins 1 3/4")	503 mg	25%	14%
Hamburger (100 g)	480 mg	24%	14%
Tomato (puree, 6 T)	426 mg	21%	12%
Banana (1 small)	370 mg	19%	11%
Peas (2/3 C)	316 mg	16%	9%
Yeast (Torula, 1 T)	205 mg	10%	6%
Parsley (1 T)	73 mg	4%	2%

There is no DRI for potassium, but 1600 to 2000 mg is the estimated minimum requirement.
Abbreviations: C, cup; T, tablespoon.

dietary and activity habits is an ongoing process. Small steps over time can help to meet goals without overwhelming changes that may not last. Behavioral modification can be as simple as assessing favorite foods, reviewing dietary intake, and making agreed-upon changes that capitalize on existing behaviors. Other behavioral techniques include food diaries, avoiding distractions during meals, not eating too rapidly (chewing more slowly, taking smaller bites, putting utensils down between bites), and reducing portions. The size of a fist is considered an adequate portion size.

Avoid and Choose Lists

The use of avoid and choose lists (**Table 5**) can educate the patient without the necessity of always counting calories. Such educational tools can help the patient achieve behavioral change and can reduce total calorie intake.

Healthy Shopping

A first rule of healthy shopping is not shopping when hungry. Too many things look good and tempting. A shopping list is also necessary. Healthy shopping lists and grocery store guides are available on the Internet.[8,9]

Restaurants

Calorie intake often increases when dining out. Patients should be encouraged to share foods, get a take-home box, and order appetizers rather than entrees. Avoidance of foods that are fried, creamed, and battered is usually in order. Selections of foods that are boiled, steamed, grilled, or baked are usually better choices. Sauces and dressings should be ordered "on the side." Order the smaller hamburger, skip the fries, and do not eat the top bun or bread slice. Drink water or a sugar-free beverage, and for dessert, have frozen yogurt or light ice cream, and consider the child's size. Ordering first can help reduce the influence of fellow diners' tempting choices.

Breakfast

Eating breakfast is one way to help control weight and increase metabolism for the day.[10,11] Eating multiple meals per day and preloading with high-fiber foods (ie, fruit or vegetables) before a meal can increase the feeling of satiety without overconsuming. The adage "never too full or too hungry" seems to work.

Nutrition Prescription

A nutrition prescription can be used to emphasize important lifestyle changes needed and help clarify to the patients pertinent instructions given to them. It can be used to help set goals and can act as a contract with the patient. Patient involvement in plan and goal setting is essential. The nutrition prescription is also useful in addressing needed change at a later date. An example is shown in **Fig. 1**.

LIFESTYLE MODIFICATION

Vegetarianism

Vegetarian diets are basically plant based, with fruits, vegetables, legumes, seeds, and nuts. There are 3 major variations of vegetarianism: Vegan (a very strict vegetarian food pattern; "pure" vegetarianism), Lacto (a vegetarian food pattern that includes milk), and Lacto-Ovo (a vegetarian food pattern that includes milk and eggs).

Vegetarian diets can be healthful when carefully planned and monitored. Well-planned vegetarian diets may improve obesity, risk of coronary heart disease, diabetes, hypertension, diverticular disease, and constipation. Vegetarian diets have potential complications including (1) vitamin B12 deficiency, (2) iron-deficiency anemia, (3) vitamin D deficiency or rickets, (4) low Omega-3 PUFAs, essential amino acids, and calcium content. A carefully planned vegetarian diet should encourage a wide variety of foods and nutritionally adequate menus with sufficient calories. Specific age groups (infant, child, pregnant, lactating, or elderly) often need close monitoring. Prevention and correction of anemia are concerns. The American Dietetic Association recommends reduction of the intake of less nutrient-dense foods, such as sweets and fatty foods and encourages choices that increase the use of whole- or unrefined grain products and a variety of nuts, seeds, legumes, fruits, and vegetables. It also recommends inclusion of good sources of vitamin C to improve iron absorption and choosing low-fat or nonfat varieties of dairy products.

Dietary Supplements

Recommendations for taking supplements include the following: avoiding mega doses and choosing supplements that provide 100% of the daily value of all the vitamins unless there is a diagnosed deficiency. The label should state "United States Pharmacopeia," indicating that the amount of nutrients listed is accurate and that it will dissolve in 60 minutes. Many supplements now have added herbs, enzymes, or amino acids that may interfere with medications such as anticoagulants. Individuals should check with their physician, pharmacist, or registered dietitian (RD) before taking other than 100% DRI.[13]

Many individuals will not meet the needed recommended levels of nutrients. A vitamin/mineral supplement that does not exceed 100% of the DRI may be helpful if an individual is

1. on a very low-calorie weight-loss diet
2. elderly and not eating as much as needed
3. a strict vegetarian
4. does not consume milk, cheese, or yogurt
5. a post-gastric bypass or lap banding patient.

Overuse of multivitamin and mineral supplements is of concern.[14,15] There is a possibility that excessive vitamin A can increase the risk of hip fractures[16] and excessive iron intake could aggravate hemochromatosis.[17] Other concerns include vitamin B12 deficiency being masked by large intakes of folate.[18] Supplementation of single nutrients can sometimes have adverse effects on the absorption and use of other nutrients and medications. Beta carotene, Vitamin A, and Vitamin E may increase mortality.[19–22] If calcium supplementation is needed, an additional calcium supplement should be taken in addition to the low amount that is in multivitamin and mineral supplements.

FAT GUARDING LEGACY AND THE "YO-YO SYNDROME"

Weight history is an important component of developing a plan for an overweight patient. A history of weight loss and regain often referred to as the "yo-yo syndrome" has direct consequences for future weight reduction and health. Self-imposed or otherwise low-calorie and starvation diets evoke a "fat guarding legacy." This starvation response is important in times of starvation, such as famine.[12] The metabolic rate drops, and efficiency of absorption often increases. An individual who undergoes a rapid decrease in caloric intake will experience a resting metabolic rate (RMR) decrease often within 24 to 36 hours. This built-in conservation of energy has a downside to those attempting weight loss. RMR may be 75 cal/h, and with subsequent "starvation" episodes, RMR may drop as low as 35 to 40 cal/h.

Table 5
Example of an "avoid and choose" list

	Choose	Go Easy	Avoid
Meat, poultry, fish, and shellfish (up to 5 oz/d)	Lean cuts of meat with fat trimmed, chicken and turkey without skin, fish	Shellfish	"Prime"-grade fatty cuts of meat, goose, duck, liver, kidneys, sausage, bacon, regular luncheon meats, hot dogs
Dairy products, Milk, yogurt, cheese, (2 or more servings/day; 3–4 for pregnant or breastfeeding women)	Skim milk, 1% milk, low-fat buttermilk, evaporated skim milk, low-fat yogurt, low-fat cottage cheese, cheeses with no more than 3 g fat per ounce	2% fat milk, yogurt, part-skim ricotta, part skim or imitation hard cheeses (like part-skim milk mozzarella), "lite" cream cheese, "lite" sour cream	Whole milk, cream, half-and-half, imitation milk products, whipped cream, custard-style yogurt, whole-milk ricotta, hard cheeses (like Swiss, American, cheddar, muenster) cream cheese, sour cream
Eggs	Egg whites, cholesterol-free egg substitutes	Egg yolks (3–4/wk)	—
Fats and oils, (approximately 5–8 teaspoons/day)	Corn, olive, canola, safflower, sesame, soybean, and sunflower oils; margarine that has liquid vegetable oil as the first listed ingredient and <2 g of saturated fat per serving	Nuts, seeds, avocados, olives, peanut oil	Saturated fat, butter, lard, bacon fat, coconut palm, and palm kernel oils

Breads, cereals, pasta, rice, dried peas, and beans (6 or more servings/day)	Most breads, water bagels, English muffins, rice cakes, low-fat crackers (like matzo, bread sticks, rye crisps, saltines); hot and cold cereals; spaghetti, macaroni, noodles, and any grain rice; dried peas and beans; plain baked potato	Store-bought pancakes, waffles, biscuits, muffins, and cornbread	Croissants, sweet rolls, Danish, doughnuts, and crackers made with saturated oils; granola-type cereals made with saturated oils; egg noodles, pasta, and rice prepared with cream, butter, or cheese sauces; scalloped potato
Fruits and vegetables (5 or more servings/day	Fresh, frozen, or dried fruits; canned fruits (watch sodium content)	Canned fruit in heavy syrup	Coconut, vegetables prepared in butter, cream, or sauce
Snacks (in very limited amounts)	Sherbet, sorbet, Italian ice, low-fat frozen yogurt, popsicles, angel food cake, fig bars, gingersnaps, low-fat jelly beans and hard candy, plain popcorn, pretzels, fruit juices, tea, coffee	Ice milk, fruit crisps and cobblers, homemade cakes, cookies, and pies prepared with unsaturated oils	Ice cream, frozen tofu, candy, chocolate, potato chips, buttered popcorn, milkshakes, frappes, floats, eggnog, store-bought pies, most store-bought frosted and pound cakes

Patients Name_______________________ Date__________

1 Food Group

	Grains (bread, cereal, rice & pasta	vegetables	Fruits	Dairy (milk, yogurt & cheese)	Meat Or meat alternatives
Recommended Daily Servings					
Your daily serving					
Additional Servings Needed:					

2 Fat, Oils & Sweets

Recommended: Use sparingly

Amount you eat *(from survey)*_______________________

3 Beverages

Recommended: Beverage should provide fluids and nutrients without excessive calories

Current beverage choices that may be a problem:_______________

4 Prescription

Your suggested dietary changes are checked below:

_____ Pre-load stomach with high fiber food and water prior to fatty meals
_____Eat more whole grain breads (2-4 grams fiber per slice), cereals (4-5 grams or more fiber per serving), rice, and pasta (3 or more grams fiber per serving)
_____Eat more vegetables
_____Eat more fruits
_____Eat more milk, yogurt and cheese
_____Eat more meat, poultry, fish, dry beans, eggs and nuts
_____Eat more low-fat meats, milk, yogurt and cheese
_____Eat fewer meats and eggs
_____Eat fewer eggs (no more than 4 whole eggs or yolks per week)
_____Eat fewer fats, oils and sweets
_____Drink fewer sweetened beverages
_____Drink less alcohol
_____Drink more water
_____Eat less salt and fewer high-sodium foods
_____Exercise 20-30 minutes/day
_____Weight goal

Other prescriptions:

Roger A. Shewmake, Ph.D., L.N.______________________

Fig. 1. Nutrition prescription.

Patients will often complain that in the past weight maintenance and control was "easier." The change in RMR is a major contributor. One effective and usually safe mechanism to protect RMR is the addition of increased physical activity, especially that which maintains and/or increases muscle mass. Lean body mass requires more energy for maintenance than that that for body fat.

ASSESSMENT OF NUTRITIONAL STATUS

Dietary Assessment

The diet history is an important prerequisite for assessing patients' nutrition status and understanding their food habits. This understanding can help the clinician work more effectively in reinforcing desired behavior and suggesting appropriate changes.

The 24-hour to 72-hour diet history (recall) is a useful tool in evaluating normal habits, usual intakes, or evidence of possible deficiencies in the diet.[23,24] The food diary is often useful to determine food intake and the factors associated with intake (time of day, location, mood, others present, etc). The person keeping the food diary is instructed to write down all foods and beverages immediately after eating. The advantages of the food recall/diary are many: (1) the patient must assume an active role, (2) the patient may for the first time begin to actually see and understand his or her own food habits, and (3) the clinician gets a good idea of the patient's lifestyle and other factors that affect food intake. Food diaries are, therefore, particularly useful in outpatient counseling for weight reduction.

Sophisticated dietary analysis tools are available to determine if nutrient and caloric intake is appropriate. Comparisons are made with standards such as the DRI and the Food Guide Pyramid, US Dietary Guidelines, and such recommendations as those of the American Heart Association and the American Diabetes Association. The information provided can assist in the development of diagnosis, plan, and goals.

Biochemical Assessment

Biochemical assessment can often indicate laboratory abnormalities, which are often the result of poor nutritional intake and/or absorption. Many obese and overweight individuals are overnourished with calories and undernourished with nutrients. Prealbumin (transthyretin) has a half-life of 2 days and has a superior sensitivity to albumin in evaluating nutritional changes.[25] The implementation of good nutritional intake may increase prealbumin levels by approximately 10 mg/L every day. A lower increase may indicate inadequate nutritional support, poor response, and a poor prognosis. Albumin has a half-life of 18 days, and current evidence does not support the use of serum albumin as a single marker of nutritional status. Albumin may respond to chronic inflammation, heart failure, liver disease, protein losing enteropathies, and nephrotic syndrome. Another very sensitive indicator of nutritional change is insulin-like growth factor I (IGF-I). IGF-I has a very short half-life of 2 to 4 hours and is a very sensitive marker. Low levels are associated with increased morbidity. C-reactive protein has not been shown as a valuable marker of nutritional status in older adults.

THE PHYSICIAN'S ROLE IN WEIGHT LOSS

A physician's advice on nutrition and lifestyle is of great importance. Patients are more likely to seek a physician's advice on nutrition than that of any other health professional. The science of healthy living needs to be made practical. A simple 3-minute discussion on a patient's weight can increase the likelihood of a patient doing anything about his or her weight by 300%. An RD or licensed nutritionist (LN) is uniquely qualified to assist patients in determining individual strategies to attain and maintain weight loss.[26] Clinics that do not have the services of an RD or LN should develop a referral pattern to help patients meet the goals the physician has prescribed.

Short and useful recommendations for dietary habits can be as simple as the following: (1) do not crash-diet, (2) eat real foods, (3) watch your portion size, and (4) eat breakfast. These 4 recommendations are based on eating sensible, well-balanced meals available from whole foods with portion control. Eating breakfast is a caloric plus in that it increases your metabolic rate and can provide nutrients needed for the day.[10,11]

Acknowledgment of the problem of obesity is the first step in appropriate care followed by addressing the issue with the patient. Many obese patients report that their physician did not bring up their weight during the course of the office visit. A 3- to 5-minute conversation during the visit with regard to weight can and, as with smoking cessation efforts, has been shown to contribute to patient behavior change. Research has shown that patients who were advised to lose weight were 3 times more likely to try than patients not advised.[27]

Many patients want to talk about weight. Patients prefer the terms "weight" or "excess weight" and dislike the terms "obesity," "fatness," and "excess fat." Patients want advice that is practical and usable for them. Patients want help setting realistic goals and information on available resources. Open the conversation by finding out if the patient is willing to talk about weight or expressing your concerns about how his or her weight affects health. Ask more questions to find out how ready a patient is to control weight.

The Physical Plant

The physician's reception area and examination room should have patient education materials and posters that may stimulate questions about a healthy lifestyle. These materials should be readily available to reinforce any discussion and provide an opportunity for the patient to learn more at a later time. The office equipment and physical layout may need an update. Scales should register more than the standard 300 lb and should be placed in a private area. Scales are now available to weigh almost any patient; they are constructed to have a minimum "step-up height," can have support handles that stabilize the patient, and are not affected by the patient's girth. Placement of the scales is also important. Larger BP cuffs and tourniquets for blood draws are usually needed. Examination tables must be anchored and able to handle heavier weights. Examination gowns can be embarrassing and should be ordered in larger sizes. Bariatric chairs that are wider and capable of handling large weights are available.

NUTRITIONAL STRATEGIES FOR WEIGHT LOSS

A number of different nutritional approaches have been employed in efforts to lose weight. These strategies fall in 3 broad categories: (1) use of dietary supplement additions to the customary diet (a discussion of weight-loss supplements is beyond the scope of this article), (2) altering the specific quality, but not directly the *quantity*, of constituent dietary components, and (3) limiting the total caloric intake. The use of dietary supplements is discussed in another article. Although recognizing that rarely any of these strategies are employed in isolation, we review the latter 2 individually.

Content-Restricted (or Enhanced) Diets

Dietary modification has long been recognized as an effective means of weight control. Clearly, weight loss occurs when total caloric intake is exceeded by total caloric expenditure. Several different strategies have been employed in an effort to accomplish this in a way that is both effective and tolerable to the individual attempting the weight loss.

One method is to increase the content of dietary fiber intake through the use of high-fiber foods. The rationale is the same as that discussed for supplements (above): higher fiber content increases the sense of satiety and decreases caloric intake. Simply increasing fruit and vegetable intake does not help with weight loss.[28] However, consuming them and other low-energy-dense foods does appear to control hunger while on a restricted energy-intake diet.[29–31] Thus, it appears that the *addition* of these foods to the menu does not result in weight loss independent of caloric restriction.

Another approach is the low-fat diet. The thought behind this approach is that since lipids contain over twice the calorie-per-gram concentration of carbohydrates or protein (9 Kcal/g vs 4 Kcal/g), limiting this component of the diet would result in satiety with fewer ingested calories and resultant weight loss. Practically speaking, however, the results of this strategy have been mixed. Some studies show that it is superior to simple calorie-restricted diets,[32,33] but others show no advantage[34,35] or even inferiority in the short term.[36] A systematic review of randomized, controlled trials found that a 10% decrease in fat calories is required for successful weight loss[37]; an aggressive reduction of dietary fat, rather than minimal modifications, is essential for this strategy to be effective. The low-fat diet appears more effective when coupled with exercise in the weight-loss program, at least in women.[38] A low-fat diet does appear to be important for long-term weight-loss maintenance.[39]

In recent years, much public attention has been focused on "low-carb" diets. The mechanism believed to underlie this approach is that the fast-release energy of carbohydrates, compared with more slowly metabolized lipids or proteins, triggers an elevated insulin response, appetite stimulation, and weight gain. A dietary change restricting carbohydrates decreases this and shifts the metabolism to lipolysis, which breaks down the body fat stores, promoting weight loss. The resultant ketosis is believed to suppress the appetite, further contributing to weight loss.[40] Other authors attribute the "metabolic advantage" instead to nonequilibrium thermodynamics of fatty acid oxidation in the presence of low carbohydrates.[41] Although these diets do result in weight loss,[42,43] most studies find their efficacy comparable to other diets,[35,44] suggesting that total caloric intake, rather than the lack of calories from carbohydrates, is responsible for the weight loss. Coincident with the majority of low-carb diets is a high-protein diet.[45] Although effective for weight loss, studies of high-protein diets have failed to identify corresponding decreases in disease risk markers, suggesting that factors beyond mere weight are important for health risk reduction.[46]

Related to the low-carbohydrate diet is the low-GI diet. GI is a measure of serum glucose response to a food relative to reference food that contains equal amounts of carbohydrate. High-GI foods are generally refined carbohydrates, whereas lower-GI foods are nonstarchy vegetables, fruits, and legumes. Similar to the low-carb approach, the prinicple is that a diet with a high GI stimulates appetite, insulin oversecretion, and weight gain. Some investigators have found that a diet with a low GI (low simple carbohydrates) is more effective for weight loss than one with a low glycemic load (low total carbohydrates),[47] whereas others have not.[48,49] In fact, *including* sugar in the diet increases the likelihood of weight loss for those consuming a low-fat diet[50]! The American Diabetes Association states that there is insufficient evidence to use GI in the long-term management of diabetes.[51,52] Clinicians should be aware that the GI of certain foods may cause spikes in blood sugar levels, especially among diabetic patients. A useful reference tool is found at www.glycemicindex.com.[53]

In summary, it appears that most content-restricted diets work short term. Convincing evidence that restricting any 1 particular dietary component is more effective for weight loss than restricting another is lacking. Perhaps the main mechanism by which weight loss is attained using these strategies is that limiting the menu choice results in decreased caloric intake simply as a function of boredom with the available culinary options.[54]

Calorie-Restricted Diets

Turning from the constituents of the diet, we now look at its magnitude; our focus shifts from quality to quantity. Given a fixed activity level, body weight is proportional to caloric intake. To lose weight, one must decrease intake. A change of 3500 calories intake correlates to 1 lb of body weight. Assuming one's caloric intake is equal to one's energy expenditure, decreasing intake by 500 cal/d yields a loss of 1 lb/wk. Naturally, this assumption may not be accurate; using the formulae in **Box 1** to estimate one's energy expenditure to arrive at a baseline caloric need is wise.[55]

Box 1
Estimating total daily energy expenditure, in calories

$$\text{Men's needs}(\pm 200 \text{ calories}) = (864 - (9.7 \times \text{age[years]})) + (\text{AC}^{*} \times (6.45 \times \text{weight[pounds]}) + (12.8 \times \text{height[inches]}))$$

$$\text{Women's needs}(\pm 160 \text{ calories}) = (387 - (3.8 \times \text{age[years]})) + (\text{AC}^{*} \times (4.95 \times \text{weight[pounds]}) + (16.8 \times \text{height[inches]}))$$

*AC = activity coefficient; Sedentary, 1.0; Low activity, 1.1; Active (walking ~7 miles/d), 1.3; Very active, 1.5.

Strict limitation of caloric intake is effective for losing weight.[56,57] Very low-calorie diets (400–800 cal/d), safely used up to 16 weeks,[58] are effective for short-term weight loss, but it is difficult to maintain the weight lost via these diets.[59,60] Indeed, weight loss is more easily maintained by exercise than solely through any dietary strategies.[61] A subset of those who engage repeatedly in hypocaloric diets actually end up weighing more than they did at their baseline; weight cycling is counterproductive and leads to more weight gain.[60,62] It appears that the repeated starvation-feeding cycles enhance energy absorption and retention during the times food is available, resulting in a higher set point for the individual's weight once caloric restriction ends. This is the "yo-yo syndrome" mentioned earlier.

Safety is a concern with these aggressive diets; below 1000 cal/d, there is a risk of micronutrient deficiencies.[63] Additionally, semistarvation diets alter serum free fatty acid, amino acid, and electrolyte levels, potentially inducing lethal arrhythmias.[64] Risk and benefits must be balanced when restricting the diet.

More modestly hypocaloric diets (reduced by 500–1000 cal/d from baseline) appear to have better long-term efficacy, with weight loss maintained out to 5 years or more.[58] In order for a calorie-restricted dietary approach to weight loss to be effective, the goals must focus on lifelong dietary modification rather than immediate, but short-term, results. Dietary consistency is important,[65] and this may aided by the use of structured meal plans.[66] Examples of behavioral modifications to facilitate decreased caloric intake are provided in **Box 2**. Consistent decreasing of portion size and energy density may be a better strategy than periodic aggressive restriction of intake.

NUTRITIONAL CONSIDERATIONS FOR OTHER WEIGHT-LOSS STRATEGIES

There are important nutritional considerations for patients who pursue other strategies, beyond mere dietary modification, for weight management. This includes those who pursue pharmacologic, surgical, or exercise-based strategies. Although these topics are covered in greater detail elsewhere in this issue, relevant nutritional points are worth brief inclusion here.

Surgical Weight Loss

Bariatric surgery (gastric restrictive surgery) is a well-established technique to help attain weight loss. Malnutrition is a risk that is associated with surgery in general, but especially bariatric surgery. Preoperative and postoperative nutritional education coupled with patient compliance can alleviate many of the nutritional deficiencies and concerns of bariatric surgery. Increased risk of specific nutrient deficiencies is associated with restrictive and malabsorptive surgery.

Box 2
Behavioral modifications

Food preparation

Preplan your meals

Learn to cook the calorie-reduced way

Include low-calorie foods at each meal

Shop when your control is highest and have a list

Mealtime

Preload your stomach with liquids and drink ample liquids during meals

Use smaller plates, bowls, glasses, and serving spoons

Do not keep serving dishes on the table

Stop eating for a minute during the meal

Leave a little food on your plate (doggy bag)

Snacking at home

Keep tempting foods out of the house

Eat 3 healthy meals a day

Brush your teeth after every meal and use mouthwash

Preplan snacks into your eating plan

Try sugar-free gum or hard candy, diet soda or fruit, when craving sweets

Exercise every day

Ask family and friends not to offer you snacks

Talk to yourself

Emotional snacking

Use relaxation exercises

Take a warm bubble bath

Listen to relaxing music

Get out of the house

The considerable decline in food consumption, changes in appetite, and decreases in absorption lead to nutritional deficiencies. Nutrition education can help the patient select more nutrient-dense foods and use appropriate supplements to avoid most deficiencies. Postsurgery education regarding diet-advancement schedules is also necessary.[67]

Nutrition education has been shown to reduce food intolerances and regurgitation and increase the ability to tolerate a wider range of solid foods. Nutrients most likely to be consumed in lower amounts and/or have lower absorption include Vitamin B12, folate, iron, thiamine (Vitamin B1), Calcium, Vitamin A, Vitamin D, Vitamin E, and Vitamin K. Macronutrient concerns also exist for protein.[68,69]

Aggressive Exercise

Efforts to maximize performance among aggressive exercisers may lead to drastic alterations in normal nutrient and caloric intake. Chronic dieting, often without appropriate nutritional education and knowledge, may lead to unrealistic dietary habits, which may lead to nutrient deficiencies and subsequent health problems. Disordered eating is of concern in many compulsive exercisers.[70,71]

Sports anemia (hypochromic microcytic transient anemia) may occur in the early stages of vigorous training programs. The destruction of red blood cells and subsequent release of hemoglobin result in decreased performance. Exercisers can benefit from nutrient- and iron-rich foods diets with adequate protein and avoiding foods that inhibit iron absorption. Overconsumption of protein, vitamin, and mineral supplements is also of concern and should be monitored.

Pharmacologic Weight Loss

The use of medications such as orlistat (Xenical and Alli) inhibits gastric and pancreatic lipase production and decreases fat absorption. Anal leakage, diarrhea, fatty stools, soft stools, increased bowel movements, and flatulence may occur, especially if higher-fat diets are consumed. Patients need to be taught about fat intake to reduce the incidence of these potential side effects. Fat-soluble vitamin absorption may be decreased and require the use of fat-soluble vitamin supplementation.[72]

SUMMARY AND RECOMMENDATIONS

Several points have emerged in the course of this article that bear summarizing. Although content-restricted/-enhanced diets work short term (strength of recommendation [SOR] = A),[33,35,42,47] evidence of long-term maintenance efficacy is sparse. There is less convincing evidence that restricting one particular dietary component is superior to restricting any of the others, that the diets are safe long term, or that the proposed mechanism is truly the means by which weight loss is mediated. Based on the available evidence, the authors cannot recommend for or against these diets for long-term weight management at this time (SOR = C).[32,54]

Decreasing the total caloric intake has consistently demonstrated efficacy in promoting weight loss (SOR = A).[56,57] Very low-calorie diets are effective short term (SOR = B),[73] although close monitoring is important to ensure safety, and it should not extend beyond 16 weeks in duration (SOR = C).[64] Maintenance of the weight loss long term appears to be better with more moderate calorie restriction (a decrease of 500–1000 cal/d from baseline intake), especially in the context of a weight-loss program that also incorporates exercise and other behavioral modifications (SOR = B).[61] Weight cycling should be avoided, as the subsequent "yo-yo syndrome" may worsen the obesity of a subgroup of patients (SOR = B).[60,62]

Finally, it is important to understand that the nutritional approach to weight loss emphasizes good overall nutritional practices, with the goal being a healthful diet; the specific amount of weight lost through its implementation is secondary.

We have learned that individuals select foods for a variety of reasons and that selection, over time, can make important contributions to our health. Good nutrition and physical activity habits can, and should, be made. These changes can be simple but not always easy. Many patients can be readily discouraged when they attempt too many changes at once. Small steps can be encouraged, perhaps through a simple "nutrition prescription," of adding 1 fruit or vegetable today or changing to 1% milk. Remind patients that living healthy is not just 1 meal or 1 day but the accumulation of small changes and these changes becoming habits over time. Behavior modification can be simply not bringing foods home that are too tempting or replacing them with better choices. "Choose don't choose" lists are often excellent tools to change behavior. The short but essential admonition to watch portions and be active can sum up basic first steps to meeting health goals.

Nutrition and diet's role in promoting health and reducing chronic disease has been well established. A healthy diet coupled with appropriate food choices is an essential component in our efforts at health promotion and disease prevention. Substantial amounts of health care resources could be saved by expanding health promotion and disease prevention programs that target dietary changes. Prevention measures, such as nutrition intervention with encouragement of physical activity, are essential in slowing down the progression of chronic disease. Nutrition and physical activity are integral parts in the improvement of health care. Such efforts can be culturally sensitive and address the specific needs of populations that are vulnerable. The National Health Promotion and Disease Prevention Objectives[74] indicate that up to 50% of disease mortality is related to changeable lifestyle factors. The Surgeon General's report states "for two out of three adult Americans who do not smoke and do not drink excessively, one personal choice seems to influence long-term health prospects more than any other: what we eat."[75]

APPENDIX

General Nutrition

- www.healthierus.gov/dietaryguidelines
- www.eatright.org
- www.nal.usda.gov/fnic

Diets

- http://www.everydiet.org/diet
- http://www.quackwatch.com/01QuackeryRelatedTopics/lcd.html

REFERENCES

1. US Department of Health and Human Services. Dietary guidelines for Americans. 2005. Available at: www.healthierus.gov/dietaryguidelines. Accessed July 21, 2008.
2. Appel LJ, Moore TJ, Obarzanek E, et al. A clinical trial of the effects of dietary patterns on blood pressure. DASH Collaborative Research Group. N Engl J Med 1997;336(16):1117–24.
3. Flatt J. The biochemistry of energy expenditure. In: Bjorntorp P, Brodoff B, editors. Obesity. New York: JB Lippincott Co.; 1988. p. 100–16.
4. Shils ME, Shike M, Ross AC, et al, editors. 50th Anniversary edition modern nutrition in health and disease. 10 edition. Baltimore (MD): Lippincott Williams & Wilkins; Wolters Kluwer Co.; 2006. p. 83.
5. Standing Committee on the Scientific Evaluation of Dietary Reference Intakes FaNB, Institute of Medicine. Dietary reference intakes for calcium, phosphorus, magnesium, vitamin D, and fluoride. Washington, DC: National Academy Press; 1997.
6. Greer FR, Krebs NF. Optimizing bone health and calcium intakes of infants, children, and adolescents. Pediatrics 2006;117(2):578–85.
7. Kidney Disease Outcomes Quality Initiative (K/DOQI) clinical practice guidelines on hypertension and antihypertensive agents in chronic kidney disease. Am J Kidney Dis 2004;43(Suppl 1):S1–290.
8. Communicating Food for Health Newsletter. Healthy shopping list. Available at: http://www.foodandhealth.com/Shop_FACTS.pdf. Accessed November 1, 2008.

9. Everyday eating: Navigating the supermarket. Available at: http://www.everydayeating.com/articlestools/article.aspx#Nutrition. Accessed November 1, 2008.
10. Greenwood JL, Stanford JB. Preventing or improving obesity by addressing specific eating patterns. J Am Board Fam Med 2008;21(2):135–40.
11. Raynor HA, Jeffery RW, Ruggiero AM, et al. Weight loss strategies associated with BMI in overweight adults with type 2 diabetes at entry into the Look AHEAD (Action for Health in Diabetes) trial. Diabetes Care 2008;31(7):1299–304.
12. Jonas S, Aronson V. The "I don't eat (but I can't lose)" weight loss program. New York: Rawson Associates; 1989.
13. Mayo Clinic. Dietary supplements: using vitamin and mineral supplements wisely. March. Available at: www.mayoclinic.com/health/supplements/NU00198. Accessed July 31, 2008.
14. Fletcher R, Fairfield K. Vitamins for chronic disease prevention in adults: clinical applications. JAMA 2002;287(23):3127–9.
15. Fletcher R, Fairfield K. Vitamins for chronic disease prevention in adults: scientific review. JAMA 2002;287(23):3116–26.
16. Johansson S, Lind PM, Hakansson H, et al. Subclinical hypervitaminosis a causes fragile bones in rats. Bone 2002;31(6):685–9.
17. Fleming DJ, Tucker KL, Jacques PF, et al. Dietary factors associated with the risk of high iron stores in the elderly Framingham Heart Study cohort. Am J Clin Nutr 2002;76(6):1375–84.
18. Carmel R. Prevalence of undiagnosed pernicious anemia in the elderly. Arch Intern Med 1996;156(10):1097–100.
19. Heck A, DeWitt B, Lukes A. Potential interactions between alternative therapies and warfarin. Am J Health Syst Pharm 2000;57(13):1221–7.
20. Mucksavage J, Chan L-N. Dietary supplement interactions with medications. In: Boullata J, Armenti V, Malone M, editors. Handbook of drug-nutrient interactions. Totawa (NJ): Humana Press; 2004. p. 217–33.
21. Anonymous. Garlic supplements can impede HIV medication. J Am Coll Surg 2002;194(2):251.
22. DeSmet P. Herbal remedies. N Engl J Med 2002;347:2046–56.
23. Persson M, Elmstahl S, Westerterp KR. Validation of a dietary record routine in geriatric patients using doubly labelled water. Eur J Clin Nutr 2000;54(10): 789–96.
24. Bingham SA, Cassidy A, Cole TJ, et al. Validation of weighed records and other methods of dietary assessment using the 24 h urine nitrogen technique and other biological markers. Br J Nutr 1995;73(4):531–50.
25. Pagana KD, Pagana TJ, editors. Mosby's manual of diagnostic and laboratory test. 2nd edition. New York: Mosby, Inc.; 2002. p. 376–8.
26. ADA. Position of the American Dietetic Association: weight management. J Am Diet Assoc 2002;102(8):1145–55.
27. South_Dakota_Health_Department. Available at: http://www.healthysd.gov/HealthProfs.html. Accessed July 31, 2008.
28. Whybrow S, Harrison CL, Mayer C, et al. Effects of added fruits and vegetables on dietary intakes and body weight in Scottish adults. Br J Nutr 2006;95(3): 496–503.
29. Ello-Martin JA, Ledikwe JH, Rolls BJ. The influence of food portion size and energy density on energy intake: implications for weight management. Am J Clin Nutr 2005;82(Suppl 1):236S–41S.

30. Ello-Martin JA, Roe LS, Ledikwe JH, et al. Dietary energy density in the treatment of obesity: a year-long trial comparing 2 weight-loss diets. Am J Clin Nutr 2007; 85(6):1465–77.
31. Rolls BJ, Roe LS, Beach AM, et al. Provision of foods differing in energy density affects long-term weight loss. Obes Res 2005;13(6):1052–60.
32. Pirozzo S, Summerbell C, Cameron C, et al. Advice on low-fat diets for obesity. Cochrane Database Syst Rev 2002;(2):CD003640.
33. Astrup A, Grunwald GK, Melanson EL, et al. The role of low-fat diets in body weight control: a meta-analysis of ad libitum dietary intervention studies. Int J Obes Relat Metab Disord 2000;24(12):1545–52.
34. Meckling KA, Sherfey R. A randomized trial of a hypocaloric high-protein diet, with and without exercise, on weight loss, fitness, and markers of the metabolic syndrome in overweight and obese women. Appl Physiol Nutr Metab 2007;32(4):743–52.
35. Nordmann AJ, Nordmann A, Briel M, et al. Effects of low-carbohydrate vs low-fat diets on weight loss and cardiovascular risk factors: a meta-analysis of randomized controlled trials. Arch Intern Med 2006;166(3):285–93.
36. Harvey-Berino J. The efficacy of dietary fat vs. total energy restriction for weight loss. Obes Res 1998;6(3):202–7.
37. Bray GA, Popkin BM. Dietary fat intake does affect obesity! Am J Clin Nutr 1998; 68(6):1157–73.
38. Dunn CL, Hannan PJ, Jeffery RW, et al. The comparative and cumulative effects of a dietary restriction and exercise on weight loss. Int J Obes (Lond) 2006;30(1):112–21.
39. Peters JC. Dietary fat and body weight control. Lipids 2003;38(2):123–7.
40. Atkins RC. Dr. Atkins' new diet revolution, new and revised edition. 3 Sub edition. New York: M.Evans; 2003.
41. Feinman RD, Fine EJ. Nonequilibrium thermodynamics and energy efficiency in weight loss diets. Theor Biol Med Model 2007;4:27.
42. Gardner CD, Kiazand A, Alhassan S, et al. Comparison of the Atkins, Zone, Ornish, and LEARN diets for change in weight and related risk factors among overweight premenopausal women: the A TO Z Weight Loss Study: a randomized trial. JAMA 2007;297(9):969–77.
43. Shai I, Schwarzfuchs D, Henkin Y, et al. Weight loss with a low-carbohydrate, Mediterranean, or low-fat diet. N Engl J Med 2008;359(3):229–41.
44. Stern L, Iqbal N, Seshadri P, et al. The effects of low-carbohydrate versus conventional weight loss diets in severely obese adults: one-year follow-up of a randomized trial. Ann Intern Med 2004;140(10):778–85.
45. Schoeller DA, Buchholz AC. Energetics of obesity and weight control: does diet composition matter? J Am Diet Assoc 2005;105(5 Suppl 1):S24–8.
46. Clifton PM, Keogh JB, Noakes M. Long-term effects of a high-protein weight-loss diet. Am J Clin Nutr 2008;87(1):23–9.
47. Thomas DE, Elliott EJ, Baur L. Low glycaemic index or low glycaemic load diets for overweight and obesity. Cochrane Database Syst Rev 2007;(3):CD005105.
48. Franz MJ. The argument against glycemic index: what are the other options? Nestle Nutr Workshop Ser Clin Perform Programme 2006;11:57–68 [discussion: 69–72].
49. Reid M, Hammersley R, Hill AJ, et al. Long-term dietary compensation for added sugar: effects of supplementary sucrose drinks over a 4-week period. Br J Nutr 2007;97(1):193–203.
50. Drummond S, Dixon K, Griffin J, et al. Weight loss on an energy-restricted, low-fat, sugar-containing diet in overweight sedentary men. Int J Food Sci Nutr 2004;55(4):279–90.

51. Alfenas R, Mattes R. Influence of glycemic index/load on glycemic response, appetite, and food intake in healthy humans. Diabetes Care 2005;28:2123–9.
52. ADA. American Diabetes Association position statement: nutrition recommendations and interventions for diabetes. Diabetes Care 2008;31(Suppl 1):S61–78.
53. Glycemic_index. Available at: www.glycemicindex.com. Accessed July 21, 2008.
54. Astrup A, Meinert Larsen T, Harper A. Atkins and other low-carbohydrate diets: hoax or an effective tool for weight loss? Lancet 2004;364(9437):897–9.
55. Heymsfield SB, Harp JB, Rowell PN, et al. How much may I eat? Calorie estimates based upon energy expenditure prediction equations. Obes Rev 2006;7(4): 361–70.
56. Freedman MR, King J, Kennedy E. Popular diets: a scientific review. Obes Res 2001;9(Suppl 1):1S–40S.
57. Clinical guidelines on the identification, evaluation, and treatment of overweight and obesity in adults–the evidence report. National Institutes of Health. Obes Res 1998;6(Suppl 2):51S–209S.
58. Strychar I. Diet in the management of weight loss. CMAJ 2006;174(1):56–63.
59. Mann T, Tomiyama AJ, Westling E, et al. Medicare's search for effective obesity treatments: diets are not the answer. Am Psychol 2007;62(3):220–33.
60. Amigo I, Fernandez C. Effects of diets and their role in weight control. Psychol Health Med 2007;12(3):321–7.
61. King AC, Frey-Hewitt B, Dreon DM, et al. Diet vs exercise in weight maintenance. The effects of minimal intervention strategies on long-term outcomes in men. Arch Intern Med 1989;149(12):2741–6.
62. Field AE, Manson JE, Taylor CB, et al. Association of weight change, weight control practices, and weight cycling among women in the Nurses' Health Study II. Int J Obes Relat Metab Disord 2004;28(9):1134–42.
63. Hainer V, Toplak H, Mitrakou A. Treatment modalities of obesity: what fits whom? Diabetes Care 2008;31(Suppl 2):S269–77.
64. Fisler JS. Cardiac effects of starvation and semistarvation diets: safety and mechanisms of action. Am J Clin Nutr 1992;56(Suppl 1):230S–4S.
65. Gorin AA, Phelan S, Wing RR, et al. Promoting long-term weight control: does dieting consistency matter? Int J Obes Relat Metab Disord 2004;28(2): 278–81.
66. Flechtner-Mors M, Ditschuneit HH, Johnson TD, et al. Metabolic and weight loss effects of long-term dietary intervention in obese patients: four-year results. Obes Res 2000;8(5):399–402.
67. Elliot K. Nutritional considerations after bariatric surgery. Crit Care Nurs Q 2003; 26(2):133–8.
68. Cooper P, Brearley L, Jamieson A, et al. Nutritional consequences of modified vertical gastroplasty in obese subjects. Int J Obes 1999;23:382–8.
69. Bano G, Rodin D, Pazianas M, et al. Reduced bone mineral density after surgical treatment for obesity. Int J Obes 1999;23:361–5.
70. Beals KA, Manore MM. Nutritional status of female athletes with subclinical eating disorders. J Am Diet Assoc 1998;98(4):419–25.
71. Pugliese MT, Lifshitz F, Grad G, et al. Fear of obesity. A cause of short stature and delayed puberty. N Engl J Med 1983;309(9):513–8.
72. Escott-Stump S. Nutrition and diagnosis - related care. 5th edition. Philadelphia: Lippincott Williams & Wilkins; 2002.
73. Flynn TJ, Walsh MF. Thirty-month evaluation of a popular very-low-calorie diet program. Arch Fam Med 1993;2(10):1042–8.

74. US Department of Health and Human Services. Healthy People 2000: National Health Promotion and Disease Prevention Objectives. US Department of Health and Human Services; 1990.
75. US Department of Health and Human Services. The Surgeon General's Report on Nutrition and Health: US Department of Health and Human Services; 1998.

Exercise and Obesity

Douglas M. Okay, MD*, Paul V. Jackson, MD*, Marek Marcinkiewicz, MD,
M. Novella Papino, MD

KEYWORDS

• Exercise • BMI • Obesity • Physical activity • Overweight

Obesity is a chronic disease associated with increased mortality, which is characterized by an excess of subcutaneous fat in proportion to lean body mass and affects almost every organ and tissue of the body. Excess fat accumulation is associated with hypertrophy and hyperplasia of adipose tissue cells. Obesity is defined in various ways, such as absolute weight, weight-height ratio, distribution of subcutaneous fat, waist-hip ratio, and by societal and esthetic norms. The most popular clinical definition, based on body mass index (BMI) determined by dividing weight in kilograms by height^2 in meters, categorizes a person as overweight when the BMI is 25 to 29.9 kg/m^2 and obese when the BMI is greater than or equal to 30 kg/m^2.[1] BMI is highly correlated with percent body fat; however, it does not provide precise information about body composition.[2] Therefore, at any given BMI, individuals may vary in their actual amount of body fat. Epidemiologic data point toward an increasing trend in the prevalence of overweight and obesity.[1] Because of the high prevalence, interventions for the prevention and treatment of overweight and obesity in its various forms have become of paramount importance in decreasing morbidity and mortality in the general population.

COMORBIDITIES OF OVERWEIGHT AND OBESITY

Overweight and obesity are associated with numerous chronic conditions including hypertension, type 2 diabetes mellitus, and coronary artery disease.[3] Type 2 diabetes is strongly associated with overweight and obesity predisposing to insulin resistance. Association between excess body weight (BW)/obesity and fitness level in individuals with type 2 diabetes is presented in **Fig. 1**.

Hypertension in obese patients is more prevalent than it is in the general population. The association between increased blood pressure and overweight and obesity has been shown in both cross-sectional and longitudinal studies, but the exact mechanism responsible for the association remains unknown.[4] Dyslipidemia associated with obesity is characterized by increased levels of triglycerides (TG), increased level of low-density lipoprotein cholesterol (LDL-C), and decreased high-density lipoprotein

St. Francis Family Medicine Residency Program, 13450 Hull Street Road, Midlothian, VA 23112, USA
* Corresponding author.
E-mail addresses: douglas_okay@bshsi.org (D.M. Okay); paul_jackson@bshsi.org (P.V. Jackson).

Prim Care Clin Office Pract 36 (2009) 379–393
doi:10.1016/j.pop.2009.01.008 **primarycare.theclinics.com**
0095-4543/09/$ – see front matter

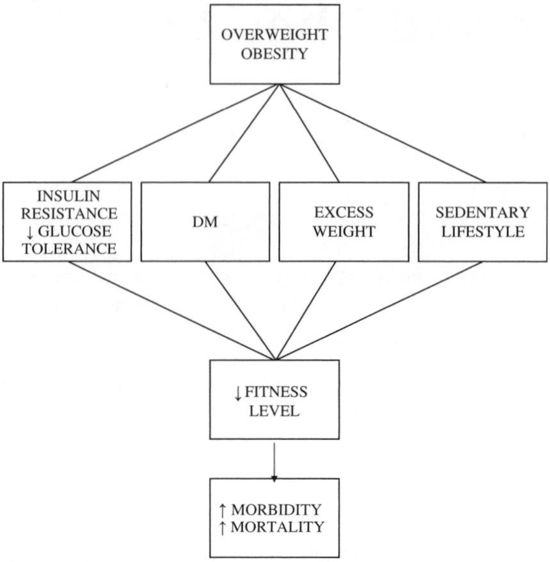

Fig. 1. Relationship of fitness and health. (*Data from* Refs. [66–69].)

cholesterol (HDL-C). In addition, qualitative changes in the size of LDL particles, with an increase in the number of more atherogenic, small, dense particles known as low-density lipoprotein subclass phenotype B (LDL-B), are associated with increased risk of coronary heart disease (CHD) and linked to an increase in BMI and waist-hip ratio.[5] Obesity has also been found to have higher oxidative stress levels after exercise, as measured by lipid peroxidation, compared with those of nonobese subjects.[6] The independent effect of obesity on CHD has been difficult to verify; however, obesity does enhance the risk of hypertension, dyslipidemia, and diabetes mellitus, well-known risk factors for CHD.[7]

Excess BW is a powerful predictor of radiographically confirmed osteoarthritis (OA) of the knee in middle-aged women and a modest predictor of OA of distal interphalangeal and carpometacarpal joints. Every 5 kg of weight gain increases the risk of knee arthritis by 35%.[8] Obese patients experience ground-reaction forces at the knees approximately 60% greater than do normal weight patients during walking. Reduction in ground-reaction forces for obese subjects occurs with walking at a slower pace. In addition, a slower walking speed produces greater energy expenditure.[9] These findings suggest that physiologic and biomechanical differences found in obese patients should be considered when making exercise recommendations. To date, no such recommendations specifically for obese patients exist that take these factors into account. Obesity also increases the risk of OA in non–weight-bearing joints, suggesting that the link between obesity and OA involves complex interactions of pathologic changes in biomechanical and physiologic factors at multiple levels.[10]

Excess BW is associated with many other medical conditions.

BENEFITS OF EXERCISE IN OVERWEIGHT AND OBESE PATIENTS

Exercise is one of the most important components of the overall approach to treating obesity. When performed regularly and properly, exercise has a powerful protective effect against obesity comorbidities. Physical activity not only contributes to an increased energy expenditure and fat loss but also protects against the loss of lean body mass, improves cardiorespiratory fitness, reduces obesity-related cardiometabolic health risks, and evokes sensations of well-being (**Box 1**).[11] Therefore, exercise may also be important for eliciting health benefits that are independent of reductions in BW. One study discovered that low cardiorespiratory fitness is a strong and independent predictor of cardiovascular disease (CVD) and all-cause mortality and of comparable importance with that of diabetes mellitus and other CVD risk factors.[12] Higher levels of cardiorespiratory fitness are associated with reductions in mortality from CVD. Overweight adults with the highest level of fitness have a lower risk of CVD than that of individuals who are at an optimal BW but with low level of cardiovascular fitness.

Evidence supports an inverse association between physical fitness and various CVD risk factors.[13] In particular, exercise improves postprandial glucose metabolism and insulin resistance in subjects with impaired glucose tolerance who adopt a relatively high level of physical activity.[14] Kelley and colleagues[14] observed improvements in total cholesterol (2%), HDL-C (3%), and TG (9%), and a trend for a decrease in LDL-C (3%) in men 18 years of age and older performing aerobic exercise. Being overweight and having a sedentary lifestyle are associated with elevated blood pressure values in the elderly, and the first step in the therapy should be behavioral measures

Box 1
Benefits of exercise in overweight and obesity

Somatic

Cardiovascular

- Improved cardiovascular performance
- Decreased myocardial oxygen demand
- Slowing of atherosclerosis
- Blood pressure reduction
- Increased peripheral blood flow

Metabolic

- Improved lipid profile
- Decreased risk of type 2 diabetes
- Reduction of truncal obesity
- Increase of basic metabolic rate

Reduction in the risk of cancer (reproductive, colon)

Reduction in the risk of osteoporosis and OA

Symptomatic and functional improvement in patient with COPD

Psychological

Improved self-image

Decreased anxiety

Improvement of symptoms in patients with depression

Abbreviation: COPD, chronic obstructive pulmonary disease.
Data from Refs.[26,70–74].

including a low-fat, low-calorie diet, increased physical activity, psychosocial stress management, and social support.[15] Self-monitoring of weight and dietary intake combined with consistent eating patterns, including regularly eating breakfast, are also important steps in behavioral management. Even individuals who have difficulty reducing their BW benefit with improvement in CVD risk factors by performing regular exercise, provided the volume and intensity of the exercise are sufficient.[16]

EXERCISE-RELATED CLINICAL INTERVENTIONS IN WEIGHT MANAGEMENT PROGRAMS

Short-Term Interventions (6 Months or Less)

Exercise has become one of the most important components of the overall approach to treating obesity; however, conflicting data on the efficacy of exercise compared with that of other interventions exist. Common features of weight reduction programs incorporating exercise into long- and short-term interventions find clinically significant benefits immediately after implementation and continued benefit for up to 1 year.[17,18] Little is known about the predominant goals, methods, and durations of weight-loss attempts in the general population. Attempted weight loss is a common behavior, regardless of age, gender, or ethnicity, and in a given year, approximately 25% of men and 40% of women try to lose weight. Among men, a higher percentage of Hispanics (31%) attempt weight loss than Caucasians (25%) or African Americans (23%).[19]

Low rates of nonbasal components of energy expenditure, including energy expended in physical activity and the thermagenic effect of food, are factors for obesity.[20] One study noted that a complex relationship of food intake and BW to the duration of exercise exists; low-duration exercise leads to slightly decreased food intake, whereas increased length of exercise is accompanied by an increased food intake and prevention of weight reduction.[21,22] In short-term interventions, restriction of calories to 1,200/d has a more pronounced effect on weight loss than that of exercise alone. However, an exercise program lasting 12 weeks and consisting of physical activity 5 d/wk, with 30 minutes of walking/running, when added to the dietary restrictions helps to consolidate weight loss achieved by a calorie-restrictive diet. For males, exercise-related BW loss and fat weight loss are minimal (2.7% and 5%, respectively), and similarly, in females, BW and fat weight loss are 2.6% and 4%, respectively. In both sexes, exercise increases maximal aerobic power [VO_2max (L/min)] to a greater extent compared with that by the diet (14% vs 2%, respectively, $P<.05$).[22]

Studies using rigorous control of individual energy intake and expenditure show 8% weight loss by daily physical activity alone. Brisk walking or light jogging on a motorized treadmill, expending an additional 700 kcal/d without caloric restriction for a duration of the 12-week period substantially reduces obesity, particularly abdominal obesity, and insulin resistance in men. Exercise without weight loss reduces abdominal fat and prevents further weight gain.[22,23] Weight loss has also been maintained a year after short-term interventions.[24,25]

Long-Term Interventions (More than 6 Months)

Long-term weight-loss maintenance is a highly complex issue encompassing increased exercise, nutritional sophistication, and self-monitoring; assuming responsibility for the need to lose weight; and developing participant's own diets, exercise, and maintenance plans.[24] The main reasons for weight regain observed after initial weight loss remain unknown. Using a combination of diet plus exercise to both lose weight and maintain weight loss is an important strategy. Long-term maintenance of weight loss is facilitated by regular physical activity.[26]

Some studies suggest that acquired initial weight loss tends to be maintained over time.[27] The growing body of literature supports the role of exercise in improving long-term maintenance of weight loss. On the contrary, Curioni and Lourenco[18] observed that initial weight loss, despite attempts at diet and/or exercise, is difficult to sustain. Weight regain still approaches 50% over long-term maintenance with diet and/or exercise, but programs including both exercise and diet produce greater weight loss than that with diet alone in obese and overweight individuals soon after the intervention period and after 1 year of follow-up. A systematic review including observational studies and randomized, controlled trials concluded that an increase in energy expenditure of physical activity of approximately 1,500 to 2,000 kcal/wk is associated with improved weight maintenance.[28]

Adherence to a prescribed exercise program remains a big challenge. Before new methods to improve exercise adherence are found, the role of prescribed physical activity in prevention of weight gain remains modest.[28] Counseling on exercise and behavioral interventions results in small to moderate degrees of sustained weight loss (3–5 kg) during at least 1 year.[29] Counseling for physical activity leads to weight loss of 2% to 3% and reduced abdominal fat. A combination of diet and physical activity counseling produces greater reduction of weight and abdominal fat than that with either approach alone.[29]

Walking is one of the most prevalent, advocated, and beneficial forms of leisure-time physical activity. Pedometers capture changes in lifestyle ambulatory behaviors that are not typically considered exercise but in fact help to increase energy expenditure. One meta-analysis study concluded that pedometer-based walking programs result in a modest amount of weight loss.[30] Other studies have found similar results that including a pedometer with brief and frequent physician counseling of sedentary patients helps patients increase their ambulatory activity and improve weight management programs.[31]

During a 5-year weight-loss maintenance study, on average, the obese individuals maintained weight losses of about 3.2% less than initial BW and successfully maintained a weight loss averaging 23.4% of their initial weight loss at 5 years.[32] Although the net weight loss maintained during this study was only about 1% of the initial BW of the participants, the groups with higher exercise amounts maintained their weight loss more successfully than those with lower amounts of physical activity after 2 to 3.3 years.[32]

A formula-based very-low-calorie diet (VLCD) program combined with exercise achieves medically significant weight loss of 10% by 90% of patients.[33] However, BW loss is maintained by only 33% of participants. Exercisers maintain more than twice as much weight loss as nonexercisers. VLCD programs can be effective in maintaining a medically significant weight loss in some patients at 30 months after program entry. Longer attendance and regular exercise help weight maintenance. The high costs of the program and the rate of weight regain indicate the need to find a more affordable and effective strategy for weight loss and maintenance.[33] Hartman reports similar results when evaluating 102 obese subjects for 2 to 3 years after treatment in a combined behavior therapy and VLCD program.[34] Average weight loss after VLCD was 27.2 kg; average weight loss at follow-up was 11.3 kg. Subjects who reported high levels of exercise were more successful in maintaining weight loss (17.5 kg at follow-up) than were those who exercised only moderately (9.3 kg) or not at all (5.6 kg). Enrolling in a weight-loss maintenance program also minimized weight regain. Subjects who participated in maintenance for more than 8 months sustained more average weight loss at follow-up (19.1 kg) than did subjects who participated for 8 months or less (10.6 kg) or subjects who did not participate in maintenance (6.6 kg).[34] The presented results highlight the importance of physical activity in weight management programs.

PHYSICAL ACTIVITY IN THE TREATMENT OF OBESITY

Using epidemiologic, clinical, and laboratory methods, different expert committees (NHLBI Obesity Education Initiative Expert Panel on the Identification, Evaluation, and Treatment of Overweight and Obesity in Adults; US Preventive Services Task Force; American College of Sports Medicine [ACSM]; Council on Sports Medicine and Fitness; Council of School Health; US Department of Health and Human Services; and US Department of Agriculture)[3,29,35–38] have independently arrived at similar conclusions about the benefits of physical activity with regard to chronic disease modification, prevention, and reducing BW. The minimal amount of accumulated physical activity generally recommended to achieve a degree of protection from chronic diseases (ie, 30 min/d) is insufficient for most persons to maintain BW in the desirable BMI range (18.5–24.9 kg/m^2). The equivalent of 60 minutes of accumulated physical activity each day is required for most persons to prevent undesirable body fat accretion.[39] In an overweight and obese patient population, the most effective algorithm for the assessment and stepwise management of the overweight or obese adult treatments involves combining and matching strategies to the characteristics of the patient. The most popular strategies are (1) weight maintenance and prevention of weight regain, (2) pharmacotherapy, and (3) bariatric surgery. Weight maintenance and prevention of weight regain are based on combined physical activity, nutrition therapy, and cognitive-behavior therapy.[40] A key component of the effective treatment consists of immediate weight loss and long-term weight-loss maintenance.[41] The initial goal of weight-loss therapy is to reduce BW by approximately 10% from baseline within 6 months of therapy. For patients with BMIs in the 27 to 35 range, a decrease of 300 to 500 kcal/d results in weight losses of about 0.23 to 0.45 kg/wk and a 10% loss in 6 months (**Table 1**). For more severely obese patients with BMIs greater than 35 kg/m^2, deficits of up to 500 to 1,000 kcal/d lead to weight losses of about 0.45 to 0.90 kg/wk and a 10% weight loss in 6 months. Weight loss at the rate of 0.45 to 0.90 kg/wk occurs safely for up to 6 months. After 6 months, the rate of weight loss usually declines and weight plateaus because of a lesser energy expenditure at the lower weight.[3] Long-term management of weight-loss maintenance requires further adjustment of the diet and physical activity prescriptions.[3]

An increase in physical activity is an important component of weight-loss therapy. Some goals of physical activity prescriptions in obesity management are to improve cardiovascular function and muscular efficiency. The cornerstone of training for fitness is aerobic exercise using large muscle groups in continuous rhythmic activity for

Table 1
BMI, caloric restriction/expended, and expected weight loss

BMI (kg/m^2)	Calorie Restriction (kcal/d)	Weight Loss (kg/wk)
27–35	300–500	0.23–0.45
>35	500–1,000	0.45–0.90

Data from Expert panel on the identification, evaluation, and treatment of overweight and obesity in adults. Executive summary of the clinical guidelines on the identification, evaluation, and treatment of overweight and obesity in adults. Arch Intern Med 1998;158(17):1855–67.

prolonged periods. These activities provide isotonic exercise, whereby skeletal muscle fibers shorten in length with little change in tension. Examples include jogging, brisk walking, bicycling, swimming, cross-country skiing, rowing, and rope jumping (**Table 2**). During isotonic exercise, heart rate and cardiac output increase, but peripheral vascular resistance falls. In contrast, isometric exercise depends on very brief bursts of intense activity in which muscle tension increases with little change in fiber length, producing a marked increase in peripheral vascular resistance and blood pressure with little increase in cardiac output. Isotonic and, to some extent, isometric exercise program can be incorporated in the management of overweight and obese adults.

People with a sedentary lifestyle are more likely to be overweight or obese, but so are those who are only moderately physically active compared with the highly physically active.[42] This poses an important question: How much exercise is enough to be clinically significant in weight reduction and weight-loss maintenance? Exercise-based programs have been found to be of particular value in maintaining weight loss. According to one study, an exercise prescription for weight loss should be for a minimum of 150 minutes (2.5 hours) or 2,500 kcal/wk.[41] Using a pedometer, this equates to 70,000 steps/wk in an 80-kg person. Exercise alone is unlikely to be effective for weight loss until around 200 to 300 minutes (3.0–3.5 hours) or 3,500 kcal/wk (~90,000 steps/wk) are expended, with effects proportional to exercise volume.

Table 2
Exercises and average energy expenditure per hour for a 154-lb person

Physical Activity	Energy Expenditure (kcal/h)[a]
Moderate	
Hiking	367
Light gardening/yard work	331
Dancing	331
Golf (walking and carrying clubs)	331
Bicycling (<10 mph)	294
Walking (3.5 mph)	279
Weight lifting (general light workout)	220
Stretching	184
Vigorous	
Running/jogging (5 mph)	588
Bicycling (>10 mph)	588
Swimming (slow freestyle laps)	514
Aerobics	478
Walking (4.5 mph)	464
Heavy yard work (chopping wood)	441
Weight lifting (vigorous effort)	441
Basketball (vigorous)	441

[a] For a 154-lb individual; calories burned per hour will be higher for persons who weigh more than 154 lb and lower for persons who weigh less.[75]

Data from Office of Disease Prevention and Health Promotion, US Department of Health and Human Services. Nutrition and Your Health: Dietary Guidelines for Americans (USDA). Available at: http://www.health.gov/DIETARYGUIDELINES/dga2005/report/HTML/table_e6.htm. Accessed August 1, 2008.

Exercise for weight-loss maintenance may need to be at around 60 to 80 min/d of moderate activity (>100,000 steps/wk) combined with a hypocaloric diet.[3]

For most obese patients, exercise should be initiated slowly and the intensity increased gradually. The exercise can be performed all at one time or intermittently during the day. Initial activities may be walking or swimming at a slow pace. The patient starts by walking 30 minutes for 3 d/wk and builds to 45 minutes of more intense walking at least 5 d/wk. With this regimen, an additional expenditure of 100 to 200 kcal/d is achieved. Another study noted that people should engage in regular physical activity to promote a daily energy expenditure of at least 300 kcal/d. Individuals should choose from a variety of activities they enjoy so that they might continue the activity throughout life.[43] All adults should set a long-term goal to accumulate at least 30 minutes or more of moderate-intensity physical activity on most, and preferably, all days of the week. Walking is particularly attractive because of its safety and accessibility, but other forms of physical activity can be used.[3] Adopting lifelong habits conducive to weight control and overall health rather than temporary measures for weight loss should be emphasized. A program that encompasses regular physical activity, modest energy intake, and reduced calories has the potential to meet such a goal.[43]

An exercise prescription can be a useful tool in promoting the beneficial effects of regular physical activity on weight reduction, disease risk reduction and modification, and helping with behavioral change. A basic exercise prescription should take into account a patient's current level of physical activity and fitness as well as his or her personal goals for being more physically active. The *frequency* of exercise, *type* of exercise, *time* (duration), and *intensity* of exercise are the main components of an exercise prescription. Other reviews dedicated solely to exercise prescriptions have delineated lists of common activities and their associated metabolic equivalents (METs) and energy expenditure.[44–47] Tables such as the one at http://www.cdc.gov/nccdphp/dnpa/physical/pdf/PA_Intensity_table_2_1.pdf are useful guides to provide concrete recommendations for various types of physical activity and assessing baseline activity levels. Percentage of maximal heart rate can also be used to guide levels of exertion during exercise. By subtracting a patient's age from 220 (for men) or 226 (for women), a maximal heart rate can be calculated. Exercise that achieves between 45% to 85% of the maximal heart rate is recommended for weight loss and for cardiovascular fitness. Adjustments in intensity should be made based on a person's baseline level of fitness, with lower-intensity exercise recommended for less fit individuals. Baseline fitness levels can be measured using an individual's maximal aerobic power (VO_2max); however, this requires specialized testing that is not always available or practical. Treadmill testing using the Bruce protocol can be used to determine the maximum METs achieved as a measure of fitness. Alternatively, heart rate at maximal exertion can be used to estimate VO_2max. The ACSM Guidelines for Exercise Testing and Prescription is a valuable reference for helping guide patients in the initial phase and the progression of an exercise program.[48] In addition to aerobic forms of exercise, an exercise prescription should contain recommendations for resistance training and flexibility training.[49] These latter 2 activities should be engaged in at least twice a week as part of a comprehensive exercise program.[44] For the purpose of reducing BW, the ACSM recommends a minimum weekly exercise goal of 1,000 kcal expended through physical activity and an expenditure of 2,000 kcal/wk as an optimal physical activity level.[35]

Based on available data, exercise in the treatment of obesity has shown greater benefit in attenuating some of the metabolic and physiologic consequences of obesity than that in reducing weight, especially in terms of sustained weight loss.

EXERCISE AND THE GERIATRIC POPULATION

The relationship between an individual's weight, health, and age is not clear. Studies of all-cause mortality have shown different, and sometimes conflicting, evidence when relating weight to age. Weight loss in older individuals may be associated with an increase in all-cause mortality as well as other negative effects. So how should physicians advise their patients regarding weight and exercise as they age? Most physicians and patients agree that maintaining a healthful BW and level of activity is important for people of all ages. However, how should one define a "healthful" BW? The most widely used gauge of BW is the BMI. Other measures of obesity, such as waist circumference or waist-to-hip ratio, have been used, but the US Preventative Services Task Force has supported the use of BMI, because it is linked with the broadest range of health outcomes.[29] However, studies show that as people age, the BMI becomes less accurate as a guide to determining optimal weight.[50]

Many studies have tried to define the relationship between the risk of death (all-cause mortality) and weight. In studies involving older adults, being underweight or losing weight (when compared with one's early adult weight) was associated with a higher mortality.[51] Bone mineral density decreases, and bone loss in men of any weight who have weight reduction occurs.[52] Clinical obesity (BMI $\geq$30) increases mortality up to 75 years of age. After 75 years of age, however, being overweight per BMI (25–29.9) might improve survival.[53] In terms of functional capacity, obesity is related to increasing levels of disability in Americans.[54]

Based on such findings, perhaps activity level and level of fitness instead of absolute weight and BMI results should be the focus in determining a "healthful" BW for the elderly. Exercise can be initiated and maintained at virtually any age, even in the presence of chronic disease.[52] Exercise, especially resistance training such as weight lifting, builds bone density and reduces the risk of osteoporotic fracture. Exercise reduces the burden of disability, improves mentation and memory, and improves longevity.[55,56] The 1996 Surgeon General's Report on Physical Activity and Health identified the elderly as a demographic group at highest risk for inactivity. Exercise prescriptions for elderly patients have been recommended and are similar to those for younger adults. Because of differences in aerobic and functional capacity in the elderly compared with that in younger adults, an exercise prescription for the elderly often needs to begin with flexibility training, progressing to resistance training, and finally incorporating aerobic exercise. This type of progression can ameliorate changes in strength and endurance that result from reduced activity associated with aging and with chronic disease.

At the onset of aerobic activities, shorter periods of exercise of at least 10 minutes each can be performed to achieve the recommended cumulative time of exercise for a given day.[44]

EXERCISE AND OBESITY IN CHILDREN

The prevalence of childhood obesity is increasing in both developed and developing countries. Children and adolescents are less physically active today than were those of previous generations. The vast majority of obese children will grow up to be obese adults.[36] There is a similar set of comorbidities associated with obesity in the pediatric population as those associated with obesity in adults.[37] In addition, there can be consequences to still-developing bones and joints, such as slipped capital femoral epiphysis and tibia varum.[57] Obesity in children, as with adults, is associated with decreased physical activity and correlates with the amount of time spent watching television or other screen time.[36] As children age and enter adolescence, there is a trend toward decreasing physical activity levels, making treatment of childhood obesity much more urgent.[58] No clear data on the optimal "dose" of physical activity needed to reduce obesity in childhood exist. Different consensus statements and expert opinions call for varying levels of baseline physical activity. The American Academy of Pediatrics (AAP), through its Council on Sports Medicine and Fitness and Council on School Health, has recommended children and adolescents to be physically active for at least 60 min/d, which does not need to be achieved in a continuous fashion but rather may be accumulated by using smaller increments. An important part of those recommendations focuses on identifying any barriers the child, adolescent, or parent might have against increasing physical activity and in developmentally and age-appropriate sports and recreational activities. The AAP has recommended that parents become good role models by increasing their own level of physical activity.[36] Other recommendations for the amount of physical activity children should get range from 30 to 60 minutes most days of the week, to a minimum of 60 minutes every day of the week.[38,57] In children, studies of physical activity and obesity show more positive effects on metabolic disease markers, such as fasting insulin or insulin resistance, than those on weight loss itself or changes in body composition.[59,60] Aerobic exercise reduces both systolic and diastolic blood pressures in children with hypertension.[61] In a meta-analysis of childhood-obesity treatment randomized trials, there was evidence of moderate treatment effect of physical activity on adiposity, reflecting the percent body fat, but not on BMI.[62] A cluster-randomized, controlled trial of an after-school program of recreational physical activity found reduced adiposity, increased apo A-1, and decreased apo B in primary school children.[63]

Few studies have evaluated the effectiveness of community-based programs as noncurricular approaches for obesity prevention. Generally, higher attendance at an after-school activity program is associated with favorable changes in percentage body fat and fat-free mass but not in BMI.[64] In another study of a community-based program, community activity coordinators and school workers encouraged children to be more physically active by increasing the variety and opportunities for physical activity in addition to the activities currently provided as part of the school program. Noncurricular activity was increased at recess, lunchtime, and after school, with a particular focus on lifestyle-based activities, such as outdoor games, household chores, gardening, beach hikes, and children's games from different countries. Those additional extracurricular activities decreased BMI after 1 year from the time the program was implemented and children continued to have weight loss at 2 years.[65]

As seen with adults, the overall evidence from currently available studies of the impact of physical activity on obesity in children, particularly in terms of BMI, is modest at best.[37] Despite this, physical activity still remains a recommended modality in the treatment of overweight and obesity in children along with other interventions. An exercise prescription similar to that for adults appears appropriate for children older than 6 years. These prescriptions should emphasize the use of major muscle groups and engage the cardiovascular and musculoskeletal systems. Consideration should be made of the fact that children prefer more sporadic play activities and less-structured forms of exercise.[44]

FUTURE RESEARCH DIRECTIONS

Because of the paucity of consistent, high-level evidence with regard to treatment of obesity, particularly with physical activity interventions, further research is needed to develop an optimal, evidence-based approach to treat obesity. To help in this development, future research should focus on the following: treatment of obesity with special attention to long-term interventions and causes and mechanisms of overweight and obesity in relation to physical activity, abdominal fat, BW, and risk assessment methods.

In particular, many unanswered questions exist about the association of physical activity and central fat distribution in obese patients with health risks. Most of the studies show statistical association between physical activity, obesity, central fat distribution, and morbidity, but the mechanism of this association remains unknown. Therefore, more investigation is needed to describe (1) the correlation of physical activity to central fat distribution and comorbidities, (2) the genetic inheritance of the relationship between fat distribution, physical activity, and comorbidities, and (3) the impact of gender, race, intensity, and duration of exercise on fat distribution. Prospective, randomized trials are needed to show clear cause and effect and to determine how much physical activity is required to achieve weight management goals. Prospective, randomized trials are also needed to provide health care providers quantification of the exercise prescriptions required to prevent weight gain in nonobese and nonoverweight population and to prevent weight regain in overweight or obese patients who have lost weight.

SUMMARY

Physical activity is a key component in maintaining fitness throughout a person's life. Exercise has a protective effect against obesity-related comorbidities even if weight loss is not obtained. Interventions for weight loss have shown minimal effect on weight but do improve overall health in children, adolescents, and adults. More studies are needed to determine an optimal evidence-based approach to the treatment of obesity. No consensus exists on the amount of exercise needed but, at this time, providing exercise prescriptions may improve our patients' level of fitness and decrease obesity-related comorbidities.

REFERENCES

1. Flegal KM, Carroll MD, Ogden CL, et al. Prevalence and trends in obesity among US adults, 1999–2000. JAMA 2002;288(14):1723–7.
2. Wang J, Thornton JC, Russell M, et al. Asians have lower body mass index (BMI) but higher percent body fat than do whites: comparisons of anthropometric measurements. Am J Clin Nutr 1994;60(1):23–8.
3. Expert panel on the identification, evaluation, and treatment of overweight and obesity in adults. Executive summary of the clinical guidelines on the identification, evaluation, and treatment of overweight and obesity in adults. Arch Intern Med 1998;158(17):1855–67.
4. Pi-Sunyer FX. Comorbidities of overweight and obesity: current evidence and research issues. Med Sci Sports Exerc 1999;31(Suppl 11):S602–8.
5. Austin MA, Selby JV. LDL subclass phenotypes and the risk factors of the insulin resistance syndrome. Int J Obes Relat Metab Disord 1995;19(Suppl 1):S22–6.
6. Vincent HK, Morgan JW, Vincent KR. Obesity exacerbates oxidative stress levels after acute exercise. Med Sci Sports Exerc 2004;36(5):772–9.
7. Kannel WB, D'Agostino RB, Cobb JL. Effect of weight on cardiovascular disease. Am J Clin Nutr 1996;63(Suppl 3):419S–22S.
8. Hart DJ, Spector TD. The relationship of obesity, fat distribution and osteoarthritis in women in the general population: the Chingford study. J Rheumatol 1993;20(2):331–5.

9. Browning RC, Kram R. Effects of obesity on the biomechanics of walking at different speeds. Med Sci Sports Exerc 2007;39(9):1632–41.
10. Eaton CB. Obesity as a risk factor for osteoarthritis: mechanical versus metabolic. Med Health R I 2004;87(7):201–4.
11. Hainer V, Toplak H, Mitrakou A. Treatment modalities of obesity: what fits whom? Diabetes Care 2008;31(Suppl 2):S269–77.
12. Wei M, Kampert JB, Barlow CE, et al. Relationship between low cardiorespiratory fitness and mortality in normal-weight, overweight, and obese men. JAMA 1999; 282(16):1547–53.
13. Hewitt JA, Whyte GP, Moreton M, et al. The effects of a graduated aerobic exercise programme on cardiovascular disease risk factors in the NHS workplace: a randomised controlled trial. J Occup Med Toxicol 2008;3:7.
14. Roumen C, Corpeleijn E, Feskens EJ, et al. Impact of 3-year lifestyle intervention on postprandial glucose metabolism: the SLIM study. Diabet Med 2008;25: 597–605.
15. Di Mauro S, Spallina G, Leotta C, et al. The effects of caloric restriction and controlled physical exercise on hypertension in the elderly. Arch Gerontol Geriatr 1998;27:1–8.
16. Jakicic JM, Gallagher KI. Exercise considerations for the sedentary, overweight adult. Exerc Sport Sci Rev 2003;31:91–5.
17. Blonk MC, Jacobs MA, Biesheuvel EH, et al. Influences on weight loss in type 2 diabetic patients: little long-term benefit from group behaviour therapy and exercise training. Diabet Med 1994;11:449–57.
18. Curioni CC, Lourenco PM. Long-term weight loss after diet and exercise: a systematic review. Int J Obes 2005;29:1168–74.
19. Williamson DF, Serdula MK, Anda RF, et al. Weight loss attempts in adults: goals, duration, and rate of weight loss. Am J Public Health 1992;82:1251–7.
20. Schulz LO, Schoeller DA. A compilation of total daily energy expenditures and body weights in healthy adults. Am J Clin Nutr 1994;60:676–81.
21. Mayer J, Marshall NB, Vitale JJ, et al. Exercise, food intake and body weight in normal rats and genetically obese adult mice. Am J Phys 1954;177:544–8.
22. Hagan RD, Upton SJ, Wong L, et al. The effects of aerobic conditioning and/or caloric restriction in overweight men and women. Med Sci Sports Exerc 1986; 18:87–94.
23. Ross R, Dagnone D, Jones PJ, et al. Reduction in obesity and related comorbid conditions after diet-induced weight loss or exercise-induced weight loss in men. A randomized, controlled trial. Ann Intern Med 2000;133:92–103.
24. Miller WC, Koceja DM, Hamilton EJ. A meta-analysis of the past 25 years of weight loss research using diet, exercise or diet plus exercise intervention. Int J Obes Relat Metab Disord 1997;21:941–7.
25. Colvin RH, Olson SB. A descriptive analysis of men and women who have lost significant weight and are highly successful at maintaining the loss. Addict Behav 1983;8:287–95.
26. Klem ML, Wing RR, McGuire MT, et al. A descriptive study of individuals successful at long-term maintenance of substantial weight loss. Am J Clin Nutr 1997;66: 239–46.
27. Adams SO, Grady KE, Lund AK, et al. Weight loss: long-term results in an ambulatory setting. J Am Diet Assoc 1983;83:306–10.
28. Fogelholm M, Kukkonen-Harjula K. Does physical activity prevent weight gain—a systematic review. Obes Rev 2000;1:95–111.

29. McTigue KM, Harris R, Hemphill B, et al. Screening and interventions for obesity in adults: summary of the evidence for the US Preventive Services Task Force. Ann Intern Med 2003;139:933–49.
30. Richardson CR, Newton TL, Abraham JJ, et al. A meta-analysis of pedometer-based walking interventions and weight loss. Ann Fam Med 2008;6(1):69–77.
31. Stovitz SD, VanWormer JJ, Center BA, et al. Pedometers as a means to increase ambulatory activity for patients seen at a family medicine clinic. J Am Board Fam Pract 2005;18(5):335–43.
32. Anderson JW, Konz EC, Frederich RC, et al. Long-term weight-loss maintenance: a meta-analysis of US studies. Am J Clin Nutr 2001;74:579–84.
33. Flynn TJ, Walsh MF. Thirty-month evaluation of a popular very-low-calorie diet program. Arch Fam Med 1993;2:1042–8.
34. Hartman WM, Stroud M, Sweet DM, et al. Long-term maintenance of weight loss following supplemented fasting. Int J Eat Disord 1993;14:87–93.
35. Armstrong LE, Whaley MH, Brubaker PH, et al. ACSM's guidelines for exercise testing and prescription. 7th edition. Philadelphia: Lippincott Williams & Wilkins; 2005.
36. Council on Sports Medicine and Fitness, Council on School Health. Active healthy living: prevention of childhood obesity through increased physical activity. Pediatrics 2006;117:1834–42.
37. Barlow SE, Expert Committee. Expert committee recommendations regarding the prevention, assessment, and treatment of child and adolescent overweight and obesity: summary report. Pediatrics 2007;120(Suppl 4):S164–92.
38. US Department of Health and Human Services, US Department of Agriculture. Dietary Guidelines for Americans; 2005. Available at: www.health.gov/DietaryGuidelines/dga2005/document/. Accessed August 1, 2008.
39. Brooks GA, Butte NF, Rand WM, et al. Chronicle of the institute of medicine physical activity recommendation: how a physical activity recommendation came to be among dietary recommendations. Am J Clin Nutr 2004;79:921S–30S.
40. Lau DC, Obesity Canada Clinical Practice Guidelines Steering Committee and Expert Panel. Synopsis of the 2006 Canadian clinical practice guidelines on the management and prevention of obesity in adults and children. CMAJ 2007;176:1103–6.
41. Egger G. Helping patients lose weight—what works? Aust Fam Physician 2008;37:20–3.
42. Tjepkema M. Adult obesity in Canada: measured height and weight. Available at: www.statcan.gc.ca/pub/82-620-m/2005001/pdf/4224906-eng.pdf. Accessed July 31, 2008.
43. Zachwieja JJ. Exercise as treatment for obesity. Endocrinol Metab Clin North Am 1996;25:965–88.
44. Warburton DE, Nicol CW, Bredin SS. Prescribing exercise as preventive therapy. CMAJ 2006;174(7):961–74.
45. Rush SR. Exercise prescription for the treatment of medical conditions. Curr Sports Med Rep 2003;2:159–65.
46. Haskell WL, Lee IM, Pate RR, et al. Physical activity and public health: updated recommendation for adults from the American College of Sports Medicine and the American Heart Association. Med Sci Sports Exerc 2007;39(8):1423–34.
47. General Physical Activities Defined by Level of Intensity. Available at: http://www.cdc.gov/nccdphp/dnpa/physical/pdf/PA_Intensity_table_2_1.pdf. Accessed November 22, 2008.

48. Franklin BA, Whaley MH, Howley ET, editors. ACSM's guidelines for exercise testing and prescription. 6th edition. Philadelphia: Lippincott Williams & Wilkins; 2000. p. 154–62.
49. Pearce PZ. Exercise is medicine. Curr Sports Med Rep 2008;7:171–5.
50. Romero-Corral A, Somers VK, Sierra-Johnson J, et al. Accuracy of body mass index in diagnosing obesity in the adult general population. Int J Obes 2008; 32:959–66.
51. Corrada MM, Kawas CH, Mozaffar F, et al. Association of body mass index and weight change with all-cause mortality in the elderly. Am J Epidemiol 2006;163: 938–49.
52. Ensrud KE, Fullman RL, Barrett-Connor E, et al. Voluntary weight reduction in older men increases hip bone loss: the osteoporotic fractures in men study. J Clin Endocrinol Metab 2005;90:1998–2004.
53. Korbonits M. Obesity and metabolism. Preface. Front Horm Res 2008;36:ix.
54. Chen H, Guo X. Obesity and functional disability in elderly Americans. J Am Geriatr Soc 2008;56:689–94.
55. Singh MA. Exercise and aging. Clin Geriatr Med 2004;20:201–21.
56. Clarkson-Smith L, Hartley AA. Relationships between physical exercise and cognitive abilities in older adults. Psychol Aging 1989;4:183–9.
57. Carrel AL. Exercise prescription for the prevention of obesity in adolescents. Curr Sports Med Rep 2004;3:330–6.
58. Nader PR, Bradley RH, Houts RM, et al. Moderate-to-vigorous physical activity from ages 9 to 15 years. JAMA 2008;300:295–305.
59. Bell LM, Watts K, Siafarikas A, et al. Exercise alone reduces insulin resistance in obese children independently of changes in body composition. J Clin Endocrinol Metab 2007;92:4230–5.
60. Allen DB, Nemeth BA, Clark RR, et al. Fitness is a stronger predictor of fasting insulin levels than fatness in overweight male middle-school children. J Pediatr 2007;150:383–7.
61. Hansen HS, Froberg K, Hyldebrandt N, et al. A controlled study of eight months of physical training and reduction of blood pressure in children: the Odense schoolchild study. BMJ 1991;303:682–5.
62. McGovern L, Johnson JN, Paulo R, et al. Treatment of pediatric obesity: a systematic review and meta-analysis of randomized trials. J Clin Endocrinol Metab 2008; 93(12):4600–5.
63. Martinez-Vizcaino V, Salcedo Aquilar F, Franguelo Gutierrez R, et al. Assessment of an after-school physical activity program to prevent obesity among 9- to 10-year-old children: a cluster randomized trial. Int J Obes (Lond) 2008;32(1):12–22.
64. Yin Z, Moore JB, Johnson MH, et al. The Medical College of Georgia Fitkid project: the relations between program attendance and changes in outcomes in year 1. Int J Obes (Lond) 2005;29(Suppl 2):S240–5.
65. Taylor RW, McAuley KA, Barbezat W, et al. APPLE project: 2-y findings of a community-based obesity prevention program in primary school age children. Am J Clin Nutr 2007;86(3):735–42.
66. Manson JE, Skerrett PJ, Greenland P, et al. The escalating pandemics of obesity and sedentary lifestyle. A call to action for clinicians. Arch Intern Med 2004; 164(3):249–58.
67. Ugur-Altun B, Altun A, Tatli E, et al. Factors related to exercise capacity in asymptomatic middle-aged type 2 diabetic patients. Diabetes Res Clin Pract 2005; 67(2):130–6.

68. Dengel DR, Hagberg JM, Pratley RE, et al. Improvements in blood pressure, glucose metabolism, and lipoprotein lipids after aerobic exercise plus weight loss in obese, hypertensive middle-aged men. Metabolism 1998;47(9): 1075–82.
69. Uusitupa MI. Early lifestyle intervention in patients with non-insulin-dependent diabetes mellitus and impaired glucose tolerance. Annu Mediaev 1996;28(5): 445–9.
70. Warburton DE, Nicol CW, Bredin SS. Health benefits of physical activity: the evidence. CMAJ 2006;174:801–9.
71. Church TS, Earnest CP, Skinner JS, et al. Effects of different doses of physical activity on cardiorespiratory fitness among sedentary, overweight or obese postmenopausal women with elevated blood pressure: a randomized controlled trial. JAMA 2007;297:2081–91.
72. Griffin TM, Guilak F. The role of mechanical loading in the onset and progression of osteoarthritis. Exerc Sport Sci Rev 2005;33:195–200.
73. Kelley DE, Goodpaster BH. Effects of physical activity on insulin action and glucose tolerance in obesity. Med Sci Sports Exerc 1999;31:S619–23.
74. Novak M, Ahlgren C, Hammarstrom A. A life-course approach in explaining social inequity in obesity among young adult men and women. Int J Obes 2006;30: 191–200.
75. Office of Disease Prevention and Health Promotion, US Department of Health and Human Services. Nutrition and Your Health: Dietary Guidelines for Americans (USDA). Available at: http://www.health.gov/DIETARYGUIDELINES/dga2005/report/HTML/table_e6.htm. Accessed August 1, 2008.

Complementary and Alternative Therapies for Weight Loss

Terrence E. Steyer, MD[a,*], Adrienne Ables, PharmD[b]

KEYWORDS

• Obesity • Complementary therapies • Dietary supplements
• Acupuncture • Hypnosis

Complementary and alternative medicine is defined as "...the use and practice of therapies or diagnostic techniques that may not be part of any current Western health care system, culture, or society."[1] Examples of complementary therapies include acupuncture, chiropractic, herbal medicine, homeopathy, and naturopathy. This definition acknowledges that the use of complementary therapies is not part of conventional health care in the United States as it is taught today. However, evidence suggests that it is one of the fastest growing segments in health care today.

Studies have shown that 34% of the US population was using at least 1 form of complementary medicine in 1990. As mentioned here, by 1997 that number had grown to 42%. This amounts to 629 million office visits to alternative practitioners in 1997 compared with 386 million office visits to primary care providers.[1,2] In one study more specific to family medicine, 50% of patients at a family medicine center were using at least 1 complementary therapy. However, only half of them had shared this information with their family physician.[3]

With the increasing prevalence of obesity and the large number of people who are using complementary therapies, there are a large number of alternative treatments touted for weight loss. Dietary supplements are the most commonly used complementary therapy for weight loss. A recent study showed that 34% of a representative sample used a dietary supplement for weight loss sometime in their lives, and nearly 1 in 10 have done so in the past year.[4,5] These supplements may be purchased in a variety of methods, from pharmacies, groceries, discount stores, gas stations, and via mail order or the Internet. In spite of the many formulations available, there is little quantifiable evidence of safety or efficacy for the top 10 most common ingredients.[6] There is an association between the use of supplements and both lower initial body mass index (BMI) and slower age-associated weight gain.[7] Additionally, those

[a] Department of Family Medicine, Medical University of South Carolina, 9228 Medical Plaza Drive, Charleston, SC 29406, USA
[b] Spartanburg Family Medicine Residency, 853 North Church Street, Spartanburg, SC 29303, USA
* Corresponding author.
E-mail address: steyerte@musc.edu (T.E. Steyer).

Prim Care Clin Office Pract 36 (2009) 395–406
doi:10.1016/j.pop.2009.01.011 primarycare.theclinics.com
0095-4543/09/$ – see front matter

who use supplements as a part of their weight loss program are also more likely to have an adequate intake of essential nutrients when compared with those who do not take supplements.[8]

With regard to other complementary therapies, a secondary analysis of nationally representative data from the National Physical Activity and Weight Loss Survey conducted in 2002 showed that 3.3% of respondents used a complementary therapy, other than dietary supplements, to help with weight loss. The majority of these individuals used yoga for weight control, whereas smaller numbers used medication, acupuncture, massage, or martial arts.[9]

This article systematically reviews the most commonly used dietary supplements for weight loss as well as other complementary therapies that individuals may use to treat their obesity. The proposed mechanisms of supplements' actions will be discussed, which include appetite suppression, metabolism boosting (eg, "fat burners"), and inhibition of nutrient absorption (eg, "fat- or carb blockers"). Safety data are also presented when available.

DIETARY SUPPLEMENTS

Caffeine/Ephedrine/Ephedrine Alkaloids

About 80% of supplements used contain naturally occurring stimulants, such as caffeine and ephedrine.[5] The combination of caffeine and ephedrine has thermogenic properties that increase energy expenditure and promote weight loss. Numerous studies have evaluated the effects of caffeine and ephedrine on weight loss in overweight and obese subjects with the typical dose being 200 mg caffeine/20 mg ephedrine 3 times daily. Ephedrine is the primary active ingredient of herbal ephedra, also known as ma huang. In herbal products, caffeine is often derived from guarana or kola nut.

An 8-week randomized, double-blind, placebo-controlled study of 67 overweight (BMI 29–35 kg/m^2) adult subjects demonstrated that the combination of ma huang and guarana, 72 mg/240 mg/d, effectively decreased weight, with an average loss of 4 kg compared with 0.8 kg in the placebo-treated group.[10] Percentage of body fat, waist and hip circumferences, and serum triglyceride (TG) concentrations also decreased significantly more in the active treatment group. There were no differences in blood pressure or blood chemistries; however, heart rate increased significantly more in the active treatment group, 7 beats per minute (bpm). There were 8 dropouts potentially due to adverse effects in the active group (elevated blood pressure, palpitations with or without chest pain, and irritability) versus none in the placebo group.

In a 12-week study of 102 overweight/obese (BMI 30–39.9 kg/m^2), adult volunteers, subjects receiving the combination of ma huang and caffeine from kola nut lost an average of 2.1 kg compared with 0.46 kg in placebo-treated patients ($P = .002$).[11] Additionally, waist circumference decreased significantly in the active treatment group compared with that in the control group, 2.57 cm and 0.91 cm, respectively ($P = .006$). There were no significant differences between the groups in reduction of percent body fat, fat mass, total cholesterol, triglycerides, blood pressure, or pulse. There was also no difference in the occurrence of adverse events between the 2 groups. However, 1 patient in each group withdrew from the study due to elevated blood pressure. A major criticism of this study is that the active product, which was to contain 10 mg ephedra and 60 mg caffeine per caplet, contained only half of the labeled ingredients, 4.15 mg ephedra and 25.3 mg caffeine per unit, so that subjects received less than half the intended study dose.

Boozer and colleagues[12] designed a prospective, randomized, double-blind, placebo-controlled study to examine the long-term safety and efficacy of a ma huang/kola nut supplement for weight loss. About 167 healthy, adult volunteers (BMI 25–40 kg/m^2) were randomized to receive 30 mg ephedrine alkaloids/64 mg caffeine or placebo 3 times daily. At randomization, all subjects were counseled to limit dietary fat intake to 30% of calories and exercise moderately. They were also given handouts on good eating habits and a progressive exercise program. At 6 months, subjects in the herbal treatment group lost significantly more weight and body fat than that of those in the placebo group, 5.3 kg versus 2.6 kg ($P = .001$) and 4.3 kg versus 2.7 kg ($P = .020$), respectively. Other significant differences in favor of the herbal group included decreased waist and hip circumferences. Blood pressure was not significantly different between the 2 groups, but heart rate increased significantly in the herbal group and decreased in the placebo group, (+ 4 bpm vs 3 bpm). Both LDL and HDL cholesterol improved significantly in the herbal group. Blood glucose remained unchanged in the treatment group and increased by 3 mg/dL in the placebo group. There were no other significant changes or differences in blood chemistries. Dry mouth, heartburn, and insomnia were reported significantly more in the active treatment group, but dropouts due to adverse effects did not differ between the 2 groups.

Another study also examined the chronic effects of an ephedrine/caffeine mixture in adult obese adults.[13] This was an open-label continuation study of a 24-week, double-blind, randomized study of ephedrine/caffeine 20 mg/200 mg, ephedrine, caffeine or placebo 3 times daily. Subjects who had no withdrawal symptoms during the 2 weeks of study cessation and who were more than 110% of ideal body weight were included. Of the 141 patients who completed the original study, 99 completed the open-label study to week 50. Only the weight loss within the original caffeine group, 2.4 kg, was significant ($P = .01$). However, the other groups did maintain their weight loss from the original 24-week trial. Five patients dropped out of the study due to adverse effects, 2 in the ephedrine group and 3 in the caffeine group, with insomnia, nervousness, and irritability being the most common reasons. Decreases in blood glucose, TG, and total cholesterol were maintained in all groups at week 50.[14]

Finally, a meta-analysis evaluating the efficacy and safety of ephedrine for weight loss and athletic performance was performed.[15] Eligible studies had to be at least 8 weeks in duration and report weight loss outcomes and adverse effects. The authors identified 12 trials that assessed the effect of ephedrine with caffeine versus placebo for weight loss. The estimate of the rate of weight loss was 1 kg/mo more than weight loss with placebo. Seven published controlled trials assessed the combination on athletic performance, but they were not appropriate for pooled analysis due to the heterogeneity in types of exercise as well as outcome measures. About 50 trials were included in the safety assessment of ephedrine. Subjects receiving ephedrine had a 2.2 to 3.6 increased odds of psychiatric symptoms, autonomic hyperactivity, upper gastrointestinal symptoms, and palpitations.

There is sufficient evidence to support the effectiveness of up to 6 months of ephedrine/caffeine for weight loss. Side effects may preclude its use in patients with chronic cardiovascular or psychiatric illnesses.

Chromium

Chromium picolinate is advocated in both medical and lay literature for reducing body weight. Chromium is an essential trace mineral that enhances insulin activity and has shown some benefit for the control of diabetes. Picolinic acid is a naturally occurring derivative of tryptophan. Effects of chromium picolinate include an increase in lean body mass, decrease in percentage of body fat, and increase in metabolic rate.[16,17] Pittler and colleagues[18] conducted a meta-analysis on randomized, double-blind, placebo-controlled trials of chromium picolinate for reducing body weight. Trials were excluded if there were multiple interventions, that is, diet, exercise, or other medications. Ten trials (489 participants) were included in the analysis, which showed a statistically significant reduction in body weight in chromium-treated patients compared with that in placebo-treated patients (mean difference, 1.1 kg). The data also suggested a significant effect for percentage of body fat (mean difference, 1.2%) but not lean mass. Only 3 of the trials reported on adverse events, all of which demonstrated a lack of adverse events in participants receiving chromium picolinate.

Although the aforementioned meta-analysis showed a significant differential effect of chromium picolinate on body weight, the clinical relevance is debatable due to the small size of the effect. Additionally, the methodology of the included studies was variable, thus decreasing the robustness of the meta-analysis. Finally, though there were no adverse events reported in the included trials, there have been case reports of adverse effects due to chromium picolinate, including rhabdomyolysis and severe renal impairment.[19–21]

Fish Oil

Omega-3 fatty acids found in fish oil have been shown to decrease TG levels and modestly decrease blood pressure, important risk factors for cardiac disease. [22–24] The omega-3 fatty acids generally refer to docosahexanoic acid (DHA) and eicosapentanoic acid (EPA). Fish oil has been studied in overweight persons as part of a weight loss diet. Mori and colleagues[25] randomized 69 overweight (BMI >25 kg/m^2), hypertensive patients to 1 of 4 16-week treatment arms: control group, daily fish meal, energy-restricted diet, energy-restricted diet plus daily fish. The daily fish meal provided roughly 3.65 g of omega-3 fatty acids. Both energy-restricted diets resulted in an average weight loss of 5.6 kg (P<.0001); there was no significant change in the other 2 groups. TG concentrations decreased by 29% in the fish group, 26% in the energy-restricted group, and 38% in the energy-restricted plus fish group (P<.001). Although there was no independent effect of fish oil on glucose or insulin levels, the fish plus diet group had the greatest decreases, 9% and 33%, respectively. Changes in blood pressure were not reported.

Another small study examined the effects of omega-3 fatty acids with exercise on body composition and cardiovascular disease risk factors.[26] About 75 adult volunteers with BMI >25 mg/m^2 plus $\geq$1 of the following were enrolled into the study: hypertension, hypertriglyceridemia, or elevated total cholesterol. Subjects were randomized to 1 of 4 groups: fish oil (6 g), fish oil + regular physical activity, placebo oil, or placebo oil plus regular physical activity. Fish oil capsules provided 260 mg DHA and 60 mg EPA per 1-g capsule, and placebo oil was sunflower oil. The exercise groups were required to run or walk 3 times a week for 45 minutes. About 65 volunteers completed the 12-week study. Fish oil reduced TG and increased HDL concentrations significantly more than sunflower oil, 14% versus 5% and 10% versus 3%, respectively (P<.05). There were no differences in blood pressure, heart rate, and body weight or body composition in the fish oil groups.

Although fish oil supplementation cannot be recommended for weight loss, the American Heart Association recommends that everyone eat a heart healthy diet that includes at least 2 servings of fatty fish per week in addition to other foods rich in omega-3 fatty acids.[27] Fatty fish include tuna, salmon, herring, and mackerel.

Calcium Supplements

Data from the National Health and Nutrition Examination Survey has demonstrated an inverse association between relative risk of obesity and calcium intake in adults.[28] Accumulating data from observational studies indicate that a high calcium intake may reduce body weight and body fat.[29] However, few randomized trials have been conducted. Postmenopausal women enrolled in the Women's Health Initiative clinical trial (n = 36, 382) were randomized to receive 1000 mg of elemental calcium plus 400 IU of cholecalciferol or placebo daily and followed for an average of 7 years.[30] The outcome measure was change in body weight. Baseline characteristics between the 2 groups were similar. At the end of the study, women in the calcium group had a slightly but statistically significant lower risk of gaining weight than did those on the placebo group (odds ratio, .94; 95% confidence interval, 0.90–0.99). Treatment effects were seen primarily in women whose baseline calcium intakes were lass than 1200 mg daily; those whose intakes were greater than 1200 mg daily were unaffected by treatment. It is important to point out that weight loss was not an objective of this study, rather lack of postmenopausal weight gain. The only conclusion is that postmenopausal women should be advised to take in 1200 mg calcium daily.

The effect of calcium intake on body weight and composition in young girls was examined by Lorenzen and colleagues.[31] About 110 13-year-old girls were randomized to receive 500 mg of calcium carbonate or placebo daily for 1 year. There were no differences at baseline between the 2 groups in weight, percent body fat, or dietary calcium intake. Habitual dietary calcium intake was inversely associated with body fat, but calcium supplementation had no effect on weight or percentage of body fat. Notably, all of the subjects in the study were of normal weight.

There is no conclusive evidence that calcium supplementation results in weight loss.

Diacylglycerol

DG is a minor component of dietary oils and fats. It is synthesized commercially by enzyme-catalyzed esterification of glycerol with fatty acids from oils, such as canola, soybean, corn, and olive oil. Oleic, linoleic, and linolenic acids are the main fatty acid constituents of DG.[32] Because DG does not increase serum TG levels, it has been studied for both weight loss and to decrease accumulation of body fat.

Nagao and colleagues[33] enrolled 38 healthy male volunteers with a BMI of 24 kg/m^2 into a 16-week study to assess the potential health benefits of DG in comparison with TG. The test diet was given at breakfast with a daily intake of test oil, either DG or TG of 10 g, with a total daily lipid intake of 50 g/day. Body weight and BMI decreased significantly more in the DG test group (P<.01). Body fat decreased similarly in the 2 groups, but abdominal fat decreased significantly more in the DG group (P<0.05). There were no significant differences in serum lipid or glucose concentrations between the groups.

A larger randomized, double-blind study investigated the safety and efficacy of substituting 15% of dietary energy with DG-rich oil or a TG-rich oil in reducing body weight, fat mass, and intra-abdominal fat in 131 obese subjects.[34] The average BMI at baseline was 34 kg/m^2, and the mean abdominal circumference was 106 cm. About 79 participants completed the study. At the end of the 24-week study, body weight and fat mass decreased significantly more in the DG group than that in the TG group, (P<.025, .037 respectively); there was no difference in intra-abdominal fat change. Gastrointestinal complaints were the most common side effects.

Food containing DG oil may be useful as an adjunct to diet in the management of obesity. The FDA is reviewing the manufacturer's (Kao Corporation) application for Generally Recognized as Safe status for DG.

Conjugated Linoleic Acid

Conjugated linoleic acid (CLA) refers to a group of conjugated dienoic isomers of linoleic acid, including cis-9, trans-11 linoleic acid, and trans-10, cis-12 linoleic acid.

Major dietary sources of CLA are dairy products and beef. These sources usually contain more of the cis-9, trans-11 isomer in a ratio of 30to 70:1. Supplements containing CLA usually provide the 2 isomers in a 50:50 ratio.[35] There is a lot of interest in using CLA for weight loss in obesity. Small studies indicate that supplementation with CLA, 0.7 to 4.5 g/day, reduces body fat mass and improves satiety, without significant effects on body weight or serum lipids.[36–39]

The largest long-term study of CLA supplementation occurred during a 1-year period in overweight but otherwise healthy adults.[40] About 180 men and women with BMIs of 25 to 30 kg/m2 were randomly assigned to 1 of 2 forms of CLA (50:50 isomer ratio) or placebo (olive oil). The primary outcome measure was reduction in body fat mass; secondary outcomes included effects on lean body mass and adverse events. No restrictions in lifestyle or caloric intake were implemented. At 12 months, body fat mass was significantly lower in the CLA-supplemented subjects than that in those supplemented with placebo ($P<.001$), and lean body mass increased slightly with CLA versus placebo. Adverse events were equally distributed between the groups; abdominal discomfort, loose stools, and dyspepsia were most commonly reported. There were no differences in HgA_{1C} or serum lipid concentrations at 12 months.

However, other research has demonstrated that CLA supplementation increases insulin resistance and serum glucose levels in patients with abdominal obesity without significant decreases in body fat or weight.[41,42] It may also worsen endothelial function, possibly increasing risk for cardiovascular morbidity.[43] Taken together, it appears that supplementation with CLA cannot be recommended at this time for weight loss in obese patients.

Pyruvate

Pyruvic acid is a by-product of glucose metabolism. It is an alpha-keto acid, which is converted to lactic acid. Preliminary clinical research suggests that pyruvate might increase fat oxidation and improve body composition in obese persons without improvements in lipid levels.[44,45] A 6-week, double-blinded, placebo-controlled study in 26 obese individuals (BMI $\geq$25 kg/m^2) demonstrated a small but statistically significant decrease in body weight (- 1.2 kg) and body fat (- 2.5 kg) in pyruvate-treated subjects ($P<.001$).[46] Additionally, fatigue decreased and vigor significantly increased in this group compared with that in placebo.

Another group of investigators evaluated the effects of pyruvate supplementation during training on body composition and exercise capacity.[47] Twenty-three females with an average BMI of 27 kg/m^2 were randomized to calcium pyruvate 5 g or placebo 2 times daily for 30 days. All subjects were also enrolled in a 30-day resistance training and walking program. Pyruvate-treated subjects gained less weight and lost more fat than did placebo-treated subjects, but these changes were not statistically significant. There were also no differences between groups in maximal exercise responses. Notably, there was some evidence to suggest that pyruvate negated the beneficial effects of exercise on HDL values.

More evidence is needed before pyruvate can be recommended for weight loss.

Garcinia

Hydroxycitric acid comes from the fruit and rind of garcinia and is theorized to interfere with lipogenesis.[48] It is often marketed as an appetite suppressant. Two small short-term studies did not demonstrate a decrease in body weight or fat oxidation in overweight subjects compared with that with placebo.[49,50]

Heymsfield and colleagues[48] randomized 135 overweight adults (BMI 32 kg/m^2) to 1500 mg hydroxycitric acid per day or placebo in addition to a high-fiber, low-energy diet. At 12 weeks, patients in both groups lost a significant amount of weight from baseline, with no statistically significant difference between groups and no difference in body fat mass loss.

At this time, there is insufficient evidence to support the effectiveness of garcinia extract for weight loss.

Hoodia

Hoodia is a succulent herb that grows in the Kalahari Desert. It is claimed that the San Bushmen eat hoodia to stave off hunger during long hunts. A specific component of hoodia extract, P57, is thought to be responsible for appetite suppressant properties.[51] P57 was at one time licensed to Pfizer for development, which was discontinued in 2003.[52] Currently, the indigenous San peoples of South Africa own the intellectual property rights for the use of hoodia to control appetite.[53] Hoodia is currently a popular constituent of over-the-counter weight loss products. However, there are no randomized, controlled trials evaluating the effectiveness of hoodia supplements on weight loss. In addition, news reports suggest that some hoodia products sold on the Internet may not actually contain any hoodia.

Absorption-Blocking Supplements

Some absorption-blocking supplements may aid with weight loss. One example is *Phaseolus vulgaris* bean extract, which interferes with carbohydrate absorption. Users of this supplement lost more weight than did those taking a placebo in one small study.[54] Phytosterols inhibit fat absorption and lead to weight loss in animal studies although no human weight loss data are currently available.[55]

Fiber may decrease absorption by increasing gastrointestinal motility, in addition to leading to a sense of satiety as its mass displaces that of calorie-rich dietary components. Studies show that fiber's effect varies based on its solubility. Insoluble fiber has demonstrated efficacy in weight loss,[56] whereas soluble fiber[57] and chitosan[58] do not.

ALTERNATIVE FORMS OF CARE

Although supplements are the most commonly studied and used of complementary therapies for the treatment of obesity, other alternative modalities exist that may be useful in the treatment of this disease.

Acupuncture

Acupuncture is defined as, "the insertion of very fine needles (sometimes in conjunction with electrical stimulus), on the body's surface, in order to influence physiological functioning of the body."[59]

Although the exact mechanism by which acupuncture works is often unknown, the mechanism that helps to suppress appetite in patients who use acupuncture has been of interest to researchers. In 2001, Liu and colleagues[60] demonstrated in a rat model that acupuncture affected the ventromedial nucleus of the hypothalamus. In this area of the brain, rats that were stimulated with acupuncture needles demonstrated decreased levels of tyrosine and dopamine and increased levels of 5-hydroxytryptamine and 5-hydroxyindoline. In a study by Wei and Liu in 2003, levels of tryptophan and 5-hydroxyindoleacetic acid were increased, and 5- hydroxytryptamine levels were decreased in the raphe nuclei of treated rats.[61] Thus, acupuncture appears to work on neurotransmitters within the brain to suppress appetite levels and thus help with weight loss.

Clinically, 5 studies, which have been previously discussed and summarized,[62] were found in the literature that used a randomized, control approach to study the effects of acupuncture on obesity. In this research, the control group uses "sham acupuncture," the use of needles at sites other than those thought to be active for treatment of a disease. In 2 early studies, the use of acupuncture showed either modest[63] or no[64] benefit in the treatment of obesity. Three studies had more mixed results. In a study by Allison and colleagues[65] in 1995, 96 obese volunteers used permanent acupuncture devices in either their ear or their wrist (placebo.) Both groups had a small weight loss with no statistical difference between the 2 groups. A study by Shafshak in the same year used needles in 3 different points (hunger, stomach, and placebo) during 5 sessions per week for 3 weeks. The investigator then assessed compliance of each group to a 1000 kcal/d diet. Respectively, 70%, 80%, and 20% of the participants in each group were able to follow the diet.[66] In 1998, Richards and Marley conducted a randomized, control trial using a device named AcuSlim. This device, when attached to the ear, is designed to help suppress a patient's appetite. For control purposes, participants used the same device on their thumb. The active group lost 2.8 + 1.3 kg compared with the control group, which lost 0.63 + 0.25 kg. ($P<.05$).[67]

Although the evidence is conflicting, the use of acupuncture may be a useful adjuvant treatment to diet and exercise for weight loss.

Homeopathy

Homeopathy is "a system of therapy based on the concept that disease can be treated with drugs (In minute doses) thought capable of producing the same symptoms in healthy people as the disease itself."[68]

Two studies on homeopathy for the treatment of obesity have been previously identified.[69] In the first trial, *Helianthus tuberosus* D1 was used in patients with an average BMI of 28 kg/m^2. After 12 weeks, it was found that the treatment group had lost significantly more weight than that of the control group.[70] In the second study, it was found that *Thyroidinum* 30cH was no more effective than placebo when used as an appetite suppressant.[71] Based on this conflicting evidence, the use of homeopathic remedies for the treatment of obesity cannot be recommended.

Hypnosis

Hypnotherapy is "the induction of trance states and the use of therapeutic suggestion."[72]

There have been 2 meta-analyses conducted that look at the effect of hypnosis on weight loss. In a meta-analysis Kirsch and colleagues[73] compared 6 randomized, control trials, which compared cognitive-behavioral therapy alone versus cognitive-behavioral therapy with hypnosis. They concluded that adding hypnosis as an adjuvant increased the amount of weight loss. As previously described by Allison, a second group of authors found several transcription and computing errors in the Kirsch meta-analysis. Upon correcting these, it was concluded that hypnosis resulted in, at best, a small improvement in the treatment effect.[74]

Since these 2 meta-analyses have been performed, a new randomized, control trial was conducted. This study, conducted by Stradling and colleagues,[75] looked at hypnosis for stress reduction or energy-intake reduction and compared these groups to one that used dietary advice alone. This study demonstrated that all 3 groups lost 2% to 3% of their body weight at 3 months. However, by 18 months, only the group that received hypnosis for stress reduction had a significant weight loss relative to their baseline. This evidence suggests that hypnosis may be a useful treatment for obesity.

REFERENCES

1. Eisenberg DM, Kessler RC, Foster C, et al. Unconventional medicine in the United States: prevalence, costs, and patterns of use. N Engl J Med 1993;328(4): 246–52.
2. Eisenberg DM, Davis RB, Ettner SL, et al. Trends in alternative medicine use in the Unites States, 1990–92: results of a follow-up national survey. JAMA 1998; 280(18):1569–75.
3. Elder NC, Gillcrist A, Minz R. Use of alternative health care by family practice patients. Arch Fam Med 1997;6(2):181–4.
4. Pillitteri JL, Shiffman S, Rohay JM, et al. Use of dietary supplements for weight loss in the United States: results of a national survey. Obesity (Silver Spring) 2008;16(4):790–6.
5. Blanck HM, Serdula MK, Gillespie C, et al. Use of nonprescription dietary supplements for weight loss is common among Americans. J Am Diet Assoc 2007; 107(3):441–7.
6. Sharpe PA, Granner ML, Conway JM, et al. Availability of weight-loss supplements: results of an audit of retail outlets in a southeastern city. J Am Diet Assoc 2006;106(12):2045–51.
7. Nachtigal MC, Patterson RE, Stratton KL, et al. Dietary supplements and weight control in a middle-age population. J Altern Complement Med 2005;11(5):909–15.
8. Ashley JM, Herzog H, Clodfelter S, et al. Nutrient adequacy during weight loss interventions: a randomized study in women comparing the dietary intake in a meal replacement group with a traditional food group. Nutr J 2007;6:12.
9. Sharpe PA, Blanck HM, William JE, et al. Use of complementary and alternative medicine for weight control in the United States. J Altern Complement Med 2007;13(2):217–22.
10. Boozer CN, Nasser JA, Heymsfield SB, et al. An herbal supplement containing Ma Huang-Guarana for weight loss: a randomized, double-blind trial. Int J Obes 2001;25:316–24.
11. Coffey CS, Steiner D, Baker BA, et al. A randomized double-blind placebo-controlled clinical trial of a product containing ephedrine, caffeine, and other ingredients from herbal sources for treatment of overweight and obesity in the absence of lifestyle treatment. Int J Obes 2004;28:1411–9.
12. Boozer CN, Daly PA, Homel P, et al. Herbal ephedra/caffeine for weight loss: a 6-month randomized safety and efficacy trial. Int J Obes 2002;26:593–604.
13. Toubro S, Astrup A, Breum L, et al. The acute and chronic effects of ephedrine/caffeine mixtures on energy expenditure and glucose metabolism in humans. Int J Obes 1993;17:S73–7.
14. Astrup A, Breum L, Toubro S, et al. The effect and safety of an ephedrine/caffeine compound compared to ephedrine, caffeine, and placebo in obese subjects on an energy restricted diet. A double-blind trial. Int J Obes 1992;16:269–77.
15. Shekelle PG, Hardy ML, Morton SC, et al. Efficacy and safety of ephedra and ephedrine for weight loss and athletic performance: a meta-analysis. JAMA 2003;289:1537–45.
16. Anderson RA. Effects of chromium on body composition and weight loss. Nutr Rev 1998;56:266–70.
17. Anderson RA. Essentiality of chromium in humans. Sci Total Environ 1989;86: 75–81.
18. Pittler MH, Stevinson C, Ernnst E. Chromium picolinate for reducing body weight: meta-analysis of randomized trials. Int J Obes 2003;27:522–9.

19. Martin WR, Fuller R. Suspected chromium picolinate-induced rhabdomyolysis. Pharmacotherapy 1998;18:860–2.
20. Scroggie DA, Harris M, Sakai L. Rhabdomyolysis associated with nutritional supplement use. J Clin Rheumatol 2000;6:328–32.
21. Cerulli J, Grabe DW, Gauthier I, et al. Chromium picolinate toxicity. Ann Pharmacother 1998;32:428–31.
22. Harris WS. N-3 fatty acids and serum lipoproteins: human studies. Am J Clin Nutr 1997;65:1645S–54S.
23. Morris MC, Sacks F, Rosner B. Does fish oil lower blood pressure? A meta-analysis of controlled trials. Circulation 1993;88:523–33.
24. Appel LJ, Miller ER 3rd, Seidler AJ, et al. Does supplementation of diet with 'fish oil' reduce blood pressure? A meta-analysis of controlled clinical trials. Arch Intern Med 1993;153:1429–38.
25. Mori TA, Bao DQ, Burke V, et al. Dietary fish as a major component of a weight-loss diet: effect on serum lipids, glucose, and insulin metabolism in overweight hypertensive subjects [abstract]. Am J Clin Nutr 1999;70:817–25.
26. Hill AM, Buckley JD, Murphy KJ, et al. Combining fish-oil supplements with regular aerobic exercise improves body composition and cardiovascular disease risk factors. Am J Clin Nutr 2007;85:1267–74.
27. Kris-Etherton PM, Harris WS, Appel LJ, American Heart Association. Nutrition Committee. Fish consumption, fish oil, omega-3 fatty acids, and cardiovascular disease. Circulation 2002;106:2747–57.
28. Zemel MB, Shi H, Greer B, et al. Regulation of adiposity by calcium. FASEB J 2000;14:1132–8.
29. Heaney RP, Davies KM, Barger-Lux MJ. Calcium and weight: clinical studies. J Am Coll Nutr 2002;21:152S–5S.
30. Caan B, Neuhouser M, Aragaki A, et al. Calcium plus vitamin d supplementation and the risk of postmenopausal weight gain. Arch Intern Med 2007;167:893–902.
31. Lorenzen JK, Molgaard C, Michaelsen KF, et al. Calcium supplementation for 1 year does not reduce body weight or fat mass in young girls. Am J Clin Nutr 2006;83:18–23.
32. Maki KC, Davidson MH, Tsushima R, et al. Consumption of diacylglycerol oil as part of a reduced-energy diet enhances loss of body weight and fat in comparison with consumption of a triacylglycerol control oil. Am J Clin Nutr 2002;76:1230–6.
33. Nagao T, Watanabe H, Goto N, et al. Dietary diacylglycerol suppresses accumulation of body fat compared to triacylglycerol in men in a double-blind controlled trial. J Nutr 2000;130:792–7.
34. Jellin JM, Gregory PL, ed. Available at: http://www.naturaldatabase.com. Accessed August 6, 2008.
35. Wahle KW, Heys SD, Rotondo D. Conjugated linoleic acids: are they beneficial or detrimental to health? Prog Lipid Res 2004;43:553–87.
36. Blankson H, Stakkestad JA, Fagertun H, et al. Conjugated linoleic acid reduces body fat mass in overweight and obese humans. J Nutr 2000;130:2943–8.
37. Mougios V, Matsakas A, Petridou A, et al. Effect of supplementation with conjugated linoleic acid on human serum lipids and body fat. J Nutr Biochem 2001;12:585–94.
38. Smedman A, Vessby B. Conjugated linoleic acid supplementation in humans–metabolic effects. Lipids 2001;36:773–81.

39. Kamphuis MM, Lejeune MP, Saris WH, et al. Effect of conjugated linoleic acid supplementation after weight loss on appetite and food intake in overweight subjects. Eur J Clin Nutr 2003;57:1268–74.
40. Gaullier JM, Halse J, Hoye K, et al. Conjugated linoleic acid supplementation for 1 y reduces body fat mass in healthy overweight humans. Am J Clin Nutr 2004;79: 1118–25.
41. Riserus U, Arner P, Brismar K, et al. Treatment with dietary trans10cis12 conjugated linoleic acid causes isomer-specific insulin resistance in obese men with the metabolic syndrome. Diabetes Care 2002;25:1516–21.
42. Riserus U, Vessby B, Arner P, et al. Supplementation with trans10cis12-conjugated linoleic acid induces hyperproinsulinaemia in obese men: close association with impaired insulin sensitivity. Diabetologia 2004;47:1016–9.
43. Taylor JS, Williams SR, Rhys R, et al. Conjugated linoleic acid impairs endothelial function. Arterioscler Thromb Vasc Biol 2006;26(2):307–12.
44. Stanko RT, Tietze DL, Arch JE. Body composition, energy utilization, and nitrogen metabolism with a 4.25-MJ/d low-energy diet supplemented with pyruvate. Am J Clin Nutr 1992;56:630–5.
45. Stanko RT, Reynolds HR, Hoyson R, et al. Pyruvate supplementation of a low-cholesterol, low-fat diet: effects on plasma lipid concentrations and body composition in hyperlipidemic patients. Am J Clin Nutr 1994;59:423–7.
46. Kalman D, Colker CM, Wilets I, et al. The effects of pyruvate supplementation on body composition in overweight individuals. Nutrition 1999;15:337–40.
47. Koh-Banerjee PK, Ferreira MP, Greenwood M, et al. Effects of calcium pyruvate supplementation during training on body composition, exercise capacity, and metabolic responses to exercise. Nutrition 2005;21:312–9.
48. Heymsfield SB, Allison DB, Vasselli JR, et al. Garcinia cambogia (hydroxycitric acid) as a potential antiobesity agent: a randomized controlled trial. JAMA 1998;280:1596–600.
49. Kovacs EM, Westerterp-Plantenga MS, Saris WH. The effects of 2-week ingestion of (–)-hydroxycitrate and (–)-hydroxycitrate combined with medium-chain triglycerides on satiety, fat oxidation, energy expenditure and body weight. Int J Obes Relat Metab Disord 2001;25:1087–94.
50. Westerterp-Plantenga MS, Kovacs EMR. The effect of (-)-hydroxycitrate on energy intake and satiety in overweight humans. Int J Obes 2002;26:870–2.
51. Mangold T. Sampling the Kalahari cactus diet. BBC News May 30, 2003.
52. Pfizer returns rights of P57. Phytopharm Press Release July 30, 2003.
53. Anon. Protecting traditional knowledge: the San and hoodia. Bull World Health Organ 2006;84:345.
54. Celleno L, Tolaini M, D'Amore A, et al. A dietary supplement containing standardized *Phaseolus vulgaris* extract influences body composition of overweight men and women. Int J Med Sci 2007;4:45–52.
55. Looije N, Risovic V, Stewart D, et al. Disodium Ascorbyl Phytostanyl Phosphates (FM-VP4) reduces plasma cholesterol concentration, body weight and abdominal fat gain within a dietary-induced obese mouse model. J Pharm Pharm Sci 2005; 8(3):400–8.
56. Ryttig K, Tellnes G, Haegh L, et al. A dietary fibre supplement and weight maintenance after weight reduction: a randomized, double-blind, placebo-controlled long-term trial. Int J Obes 1989;13:165–71.
57. Howarth N, Saltzman E, McCrory M, et al. Fermentable and nonfermentable fiber supplements did not alter hunger, satiety or body weight in a pilot study of men and women consuming self-selected diets. J Nutr 2003;133:3141–4.

58. Mhurchu C, Dunshea-Mooij C, Bennett D, et al. Effect of chitosan on weight loss in overweight and obese individuals: a systematic review of randomized controlled trials. Obes Rev 2005;6:35–42.
59. Anonymous. Available at: http://acccupuncture.com/education/theory/acuinto.htm. Accessed October 3, 2008.
60. Liu Z, Sun F, Su J, et al. Study on action of acupuncture on the ventromedial nucleus of hypothalamus in obese rats. J Tradit Chin Med 2001;21(3):220–4.
61. Wei Q, Liu Z. Effects of acupuncture on monoamine neurotransmitters in raphe nuclei of obese rats. J Tradit Chin Med 2003;23(2):147–50.
62. Allison DB, Fontaine KR, Heshka S, et al. Alternative treatments for weight loss: a critical review. Crit Rev Food Sci Nutr 2001;41:1–28.
63. Giller RM. Auricular acupuncture and weight reduction: a controlled study. Am J Acupunct 1975;7:151–3.
64. Mok MS, Parker LN, Voina S, et al. A treatment of obesity by acupuncture. Am J Clin Nutr 1976;24:832–5.
65. Allison DB, Kreibach K, Heshka S, et al. Randomized placebo controlled-clinical trial of an auricular acu-pressure device for weight loss. Int J Obes 1995;19:653–8.
66. Shafshak TS. Electroacupuncture and exercise in body weight reduction and their application in rehabilitating patients with knee osteoarthritis. Am J Chin Med 1995;23:15–25.
67. Richards D, Marley J. Stimulation of auricular acupuncture points in weight loss. Aust Fam Physician 1998;27(S2):S73–7.
68. Anonymous. Available at: http://www.medterms.com/script/main/art.asp?articlekey=3775. Accessed October 3, 2008.
69. Pittler MH, Ernst E. Complementary therapies for reducing body weight: a systematic review. Int J Obes 2005;29:1030–8.
70. Werk W, Galland F. *Helianthus-tuberosus*-Therapie bei Ubergewicht. Therapiewoche 1994;44:34–9 [in German].
71. Schmidt JM, Ostermayr B. Does a homeopathic ultramolecular dilution of thyroidinum 30cH affect the rate of body weight reduction in fasting patients? A randomized placebo-controlled double-blind clinical trial. Homeopathy 2002;91:197–206.
72. Anonymous. Available at: http://www.medterms.com/script/main/art.asp?articlekey=10809. Accessed October 3, 2008.
73. Kirsch I, Montgomery G, Sapirstein G. Hypnosis as an adjunct to cognitive-behavioral psychotherapy: a meta-analysis. J Consult Clin Psychol 1996;63:214–20.
74. Allison DB, Faith MS. Hypnosis as an adjunct to cognitive-behavioral psychotherapy for obesity: a meta-analytical reappraisal. J Consult Clin Psychol 1996;64:513–6.
75. Stradling J, Roberts D, Wilson A, et al. Controlled trial of hypnotherapy for weight loss in patients with obstructive sleep apnea. Int J Obes Relat Metab Disord 1998;28:278–81.

Pharmacotherapy for the Obese Patient

Lori M. Dickerson, PharmD, BCPS*, Peter J. Carek, MD, MS

KEYWORDS

• Obesity • Pharmacotherapy • Orlistat
• Phentermine • Sibutramine

Obesity (body mass index [BMI] ≥30) and overweight (BMI ≥25) are the most common nutritional disorders in the United States, affecting almost two-thirds of the US population.[1] Obesity and overweight are associated with multiple coexisting conditions, some of which include hypertension, glucose intolerance, hyperlipidemia, and obstructive sleep apnea.[2]

Historically, the treatment of obesity has been extremely difficult. An efficient and beneficial treatment for obesity, which will satisfy the desires of most patients for rapid resolution and provide long-term results, is not available. As a caloric deficit of 3500 kcal is necessary to lose 1 lb of adipose tissue and most experts recommend losing no more than 1 to 2 lb/wk, weight loss is typically slow, and recidivism is very high. Therefore, obesity is a chronic medical condition, and treatment should be initiated with the expectation that long-term therapy will be needed.[3]

Early weight loss medications were proposed as short-term adjuncts to diet and exercise regimens, in the hopes that they would aid in initial weight loss and help patients reach "ideal body weight." Unfortunately, these short-term regimens were unsuccessful, and the literature contains multiple reports of failed weight loss regimens.[4–7] Currently, very few drugs are approved by the Food and Drug Administration (FDA) for the treatment of obesity in adults, and each must be used as part of a comprehensive weight loss program including diet and physical activity. These and other agents (**Table 1**) have been studied for weight loss, but all have major drawbacks and usually result in weight gain after discontinuation.[3,8–10] Attrition rates approach 30% to 40% for most weight loss medications due to side effects and a lack of efficacy.[10] Though behavioral modification incorporating dietary restrictions and appropriate exercise is the preferred treatment, the pharmacologic treatment of obesity is an area of continued research and development.

The National Institutes of Health recommend that nonpharmacologic therapies should be attempted for at least 6 months before drug therapy is considered (Strength of Recommendation [SOR] C).[11] Initial choice of a weight loss medication is empirical,

Department of Family Medicine, Medical University of South Carolina, 9228 Medical Plaza Drive, Charleston, SC 29406, USA
* Corresponding author.
E-mail address: macfarll@musc.edu (L.M. Dickerson).

Prim Care Clin Office Pract 36 (2009) 407–415
doi:10.1016/j.pop.2009.01.004 **primarycare.theclinics.com**

Table 1
Commonly studied pharmacologic agents for the treatment of obesity

Category	Medications	FDA Approved for Obesity Treatment
Adrenergic agents	Benzphetamine	Yes
	Diethylpropion	Yes
	Phendimetrazine	Yes
	Phentermine	Yes
Serotonergic agents	Dexfenfluramine	Yes
	Fenfluramine	Yes
	Fluoxetine	No
Adrenergic/serotonergic agents	Sibutramine	Yes
Lipase inhibitors	Orlistat	Yes
Antidepressants	Bupropion	No
Anticonvulsants	Zonisamide	No
	Topiramate	No
Cannabinoid antagonists	Rimonabant	No

Data from Refs.[3,8,9,23]

considering underlying medical conditions, concurrent medications, potential drug interactions, approval for long-term use, and cost. Patients without a weight loss of at least 2 kg in the first month of treatment should be reassessed, evaluating adherence to diet and exercise recommendations and considering a dosage adjustment (SOR C).[3] If weight loss is still minimal, therapy should be discontinued (SOR C). Combination therapy (ie, sibutramine plus orlistat) has not been shown to enhance weight loss, may increase side effects, and is not recommended outside clinical trials (SOR B).

When considering an initial weight loss medication or evaluating patients who have failed a weight loss regimen, it is also important to determine if the patient is taking any agents that can promote weight gain.[12] For example, psychiatric agents are commonly associated with weight gain and include antidepressants (selective serotonin reuptake inhibitors [SSRIs], tricyclic antidepressants), antipsychotics (especially clozapine, olanzapine, risperidone), anticonvulsants (valproic acid, carbamazepine, gabapentin), and lithium. Antidiabetic agents, such as insulin, sulfonylureas (glyburide, glipizide), and thiazolidinediones (rosiglitazone, pioglitazone), commonly cause weight gain. Corticosteroids, centrally acting antihypertensive agents (methyldopa, clonidine), and depomedroxyprogesterone acetate have also been associated with weight gain. Weight loss may be more successful if these agents are discontinued or substituted for more weight neutral agents (SOR C). In the case of diabetes control, therapy may be switched to a regimen that includes metformin, exenatide, or pramlinitide.[3,9] Metformin may also be used to promote weight loss in patients who gain more than 10% of their pretreatment body weight when taking antipsychotic medications (SOR A).[13]

APPETITE SUPPRESSANTS

Most appetite suppressants work by increasing norepinephrine, dopamine, serotonin, or some combination of these in the central nervous system.[3] These agents are typically classified as noradrenergic agents (ie, benzphetamine, diethylpropion, phendimetrazine, phentermine), serotonergic agents (ie, dexfenfluramine, fenfluramine, fluoxetine), or mixed noradrenergic-serotonergic agents (sibutramine).

Noradrenergic Agents

Noradrenergic agents have many of the pharmacologic properties of norepinephrine and enhance catecholamine neurotransmission, leading to increased sympathetic activity and reduced appetite. Some noradrenergic agents also affect dopaminergic receptors in the hypothalamus.[14] Amphetamine was formerly used to promote weight loss; however, due to a high abuse potential, its chemical structure was manipulated to find more suitable alternatives.[15] The resulting compounds retained the anorectic properties of amphetamine but displayed greatly reduced stimulant effects and abuse potential.[16] Of the adrenergic agents available for use, phentermine is the most commonly used in clinical practice. Phenylpropanolamine was an over-the-counter appetite suppressant, but was withdrawn from the market due to an association with hemorrhagic stroke in women.[17]

Phentermine

Phentermine (Adipex-P, Ionamin, Pro-Fast, generic) is similar to amphetamine and modulates noradrenergic neurotransmission to decrease appetite; however, it has little or no effect on dopaminergic neurotransmission, decreasing the potential for abuse.[18] In meta-analyses of short-term studies, phentermine combined with lifestyle interventions resulted in an average weight loss of 3.6 kg when compared with placebo (**Table 2**).[19,20] Historically, phentermine has been used in combination with fenfluramine (ie, "phen-fen") and achieved similar or greater weight loss than that with either agent alone.[9,21,22] Fenfluramine is no longer on the market, as discussed in the section Serotonergic Agents.

Phentermine is indicated in the management of exogenous obesity as a short-term (up to 12 weeks) adjunct in a regimen of weight reduction based on exercise, behavioral modification, and caloric restriction, for patients with an initial BMI greater than or equal to 30 kg/m^2 or greater than or equal to 27 kg/m^2 in the presence of other risk factors, such as hypertension, diabetes, or hyperlipidemia (SOR A).[23] The most common adverse effects of phentermine include dry mouth, headache, insomnia, nervousness, irritability, and constipation, which limit its continued use. Palpitations, tachycardia, and elevations in blood pressure may also occur. With continued use, tolerance develops, and phentermine becomes ineffective, with an increased risk of dependence and abuse. The use of monoamine oxidase inhibitors is contraindicated during or within 14 days of the use of phentermine, because hypertensive crisis may result. Other substances active in the central nervous system should also be used with caution. Phentermine should not be used in individuals with hyperthyroidism, glaucoma, agitated states, advanced arteriosclerosis, symptomatic cardiovascular disease, moderate-to-severe hypertension, or a history of substance abuse.

Serotonergic Agents

Serotonergic agents theoretically affect food intake by reducing food-seeking behavior and by decreasing the amount consumed at a particular meal or eating episode.[5] In addition, serotonergic drugs have been reported to increase basal metabolic rate by 100 cal/d, which may play a minor role in weight reduction.[24] Currently, no FDA-approved serotonergic agents for weight loss are available, but fluoxetine (Prozac, generic) has been studied in this realm. Fenfluramine (Pondimin) and dexfenfluramine (Redux) were voluntarily withdrawn from the market in the United States in 1997 due to the risk of valvular heart disease and pulmonary hypertension.[9,25]

Table 2
FDA-approved drugs for weight loss

Drug	Recommended Dose	Schedule IV Controlled Substance	Duration of Treatment	Mean Weight Loss Relative to Placebo	Side Effects
Orlistat	60–120 mg 3 times daily	No	Long term (studied up to 2 y)	2.89 kg	Diarrhea, flatulence with discharge, fecal urgency and incontinence, abdominal pain, dyspepsia
Phentermine	15–37.5 mg daily	Yes	Short term (12 wk)	3.6 kg	Dry mouth, headache, insomnia, nervousness, irritability, constipation, tachycardia, elevations in blood pressure
Sibutramine	10–15 mg daily	No	Long term (studied up to 2 y)	4.45 kg	Dry mouth, constipation, insomnia, tachycardia, elevations in blood pressure

Data from Refs.[8,9,20]

Fluoxetine

Fluoxetine is a highly selective SSRI that may increase energy expenditure by raising basal body temperature.[21] Though FDA approved for the treatment of depression, panic, bulimia, and obsessive-compulsive disorder, fluoxetine is not approved for weight loss. Although initial studies indicated that fluoxetine was effective in the treatment of obesity, its effectiveness for long-term weight loss has not been demonstrated.[26] For example, a recent meta-analysis found that fluoxetine (in doses of 60 mg daily) and other SSRIs enhanced weight loss in the first 6 to 12 months of a program that included calorie restriction.[20] However, after 12 months, only one-half of the studies reported sustained weight loss relative to placebo.

Adrenergic/Serotonergic Agents

Sibutramine, the only adrenergic/serotonergic agent available in the management of obesity, is a potent inhibitor of norepinephrine and serotonin reuptake and a weak inhibitor of dopamine reuptake. It is indicated for obese patients with an initial BMI greater than or equal to 30 kg/m^2 or a BMI greater than or equal to 27 kg/m^2 in the presence of other risk factors (eg, controlled hypertension, diabetes, dyslipidemia) (SOR A) (see **Table 2**).[23]

Sibutramine

Sibutramine and its metabolites are believed to have 2 mechanisms to exert their weight loss effect.[27] First, by inhibiting monoamine uptake, it suppresses appetite in a fashion similar to that of other SSRIs. Second, sibutramine may stimulate thermogenesis indirectly by activating the β_3-system in brown adipose tissue.

Initially tested for its antidepressant activity, sibutramine was found to cause weight loss in both healthy and depressed patients.[28] In 2 meta-analyses, patients receiving sibutramine for 12 months experienced 4.2 to 4.5 kg of weight loss when compared with that with placebo.[10,20] Sibutramine was associated with modest increases in heart rate and blood pressure but small improvements in high-density lipoprotein cholesterol, triglycerides, and, among diabetic patients, in glycemic control. Sustained weight loss of 4.0 kg after 2 years of treatment was documented in one trial.[29] No associations between sibutramine and cardiac valve dysfunction have been noted after treatment for an average 7.6 months.[30,31]

The recommended starting dose of sibutramine is 10 mg administered once daily with or without food. If there is inadequate weight loss, the dose may be titrated after 4 weeks to a total of 15 mg once daily. The most common adverse effects associated with the use of sibutramine are dry mouth, constipation, and insomnia.[9,23] Like adrenergic agents, it may increase blood pressure, heart rate, and cause palpitations.[8] Sibutramine should not be used with other serotonergic agents, such as SSRIs, due to the risk of serotonin syndrome [9,23]

Lipase Inhibitors

A reduction in fat intake is recommended in most weight loss diets; however, patient compliance with these diets is poor.[32] As digestive inhibitors interfere with the breakdown and digestion of dietary fat, inhibiting fat absorption from the gastrointestinal tract, these agents may have a role in creating the negative energy balance necessary for subsequent weight loss. Although inhibition of these enzymes by lipase inhibitors leads to inhibition of the digestion of dietary triglycerides and decreased cholesterol absorption, decreased absorption of fat-soluble vitamins also occurs (ie, vitamins A, D, E, and K).[5,33]

Orlistat

Orlistat (Xenical, Alli) is a potent and irreversible inhibitor of gastric and pancreatic carboxyl ester lipase. As a result, orlistat decreases the systemic absorption of dietary fat, leading to decreased absorption of calories and a decreased body weight. In addition, orlistat may inhibit the digestion of dietary triglycerides and decrease the absorption of cholesterol and fat-soluble vitamins, primarily vitamin D. Unfortunately, these mechanisms also lead to significant gastrointestinal side effects.

Early studies demonstrated a modest effect of orlistat in promoting weight loss.[34,35] In 2 meta-analyses, weight loss of 2.9 kg after 6 to 12 months of treatment was reported.[10,20] In addition, orlistat has reduced the incidence of diabetes and improved concentrations of total cholesterol and low-density lipoprotein cholesterol, blood pressure, and glycemic control in patients with diabetes.[10] Adverse effects are common and include diarrhea, flatulence with discharge, fecal incontinence, abdominal pain, and dyspepsia.

Orlistat is indicated for the management of obesity, including weight loss and maintenance of weight loss, in conjunction with a reduced caloric diet (SOR A) (see **Table 2**). As a prescription medication (Xenical), it is recommended for obese patients with an initial BMI >30 kg/m^2 or >27 kg/m^2 in the presence of other risk factors (eg, hypertension, diabetes, hyperlipidemia) at a dose of 120 mg 3 times daily with each meal containing fat (during or up to 1 hour after the meal). Over-the-counter orlistat (Alli) is indicated for weight loss in overweight adults and is recommended at a dose of 60 mg with each meal.[23] The patient should be eating a nutritionally balanced, reduced-calorie diet that contains approximately 30% of calories from fat. To prevent vitamin deficiencies, patients should be advised to take a fat-soluble vitamin supplement 2 hours before or after a dose of orlistat.[9]

OTHER POTENTIAL PHARMACOLOGIC AGENTS

Bupropion

Bupropion (Wellbutrin, Wellbutrin SR, Wellbutrin XL, generic) is an atypical antidepressant that may potentiate the feeling of satiety by inhibiting reuptake of dopamine, norepinephrine, and serotonin.[3,36] After noting weight loss in depressed patients treated with bupropion, it was studied for weight loss in obese patients. In doses of 300 to 400 mg daily, sustained release bupropion resulted in weight loss.[37] In a meta-analysis, patients receiving bupropion for 6 or 12 months lost 2.77 kg when compared with placebo.[20] Adverse events include dry mouth, insomnia, diarrhea, and constipation. Bupropion should not be used in patients with seizure disorders.[3]

Zonisamide

Zonisamide (Zonegran, generic) is a novel antiepileptic drug (AED) that has been associated with modest weight loss in patients with epilepsy.[38] When studied in patients with obesity, zonisamide (600 mg daily) was associated with a 5-kg weight loss when compared with placebo. Zonisamide is associated with dizziness, confusion, and difficulty concentrating.[23] In patients treated for epilepsy, rare adverse effects include Stevens-Johnson syndrome and increases in serum creatinine.[9]

Topiramate

Topiramate (Topamax) is another AED that has been associated with weight loss and anorexia in patients with seizure and affective disorders.[9] In a meta-analysis of 6 clinical trials at least 6 months in duration, topiramate was associated with a 6.5% weight loss when compared with placebo.[20] Unfortunately, adverse events are common with topiramate and include paresthesias, change in taste, difficulty concentrating, dizziness, and fatigue.[3,9] As noted in one study, the adverse event profile of topiramate makes it unsuitable for the treatment of obesity and diabetes.[39]

Rimonabant

Rimonabant is a selective antagonist of the cannabinoid type 1 receptor. The cannabinoid system is involved in the regulation of food intake, energy balance, and, therefore, body weight. Therefore, rimonabant is thought to regulate food intake from peripheral and central actions, leading to weight loss.[40] Although approved for obesity in parts of Europe, Mexico, and Argentina, it is currently investigational in the United States.[8] Rimonabant has not been approved by the FDA due to concerns of depression and anxiety observed in clinical trials.

From an efficacy standpoint, however, patients given rimonabant had a 4.7 kg greater weight loss after 1 year than did those patients given placebo.[10] Rimonabant was associated with improvements in cholesterol, blood pressure, and glycemic control in patients with diabetes but also increased the risk of mood disorders.

SUMMARY

Pharmacotherapeutic agents, if recommended and prescribed, should be an adjunct to a structured diet and exercise regimen in the treatment of obesity (SOR A). The expected weight loss with an antiobesity agent varies greatly depending on the compliance with a diet and exercise regimen. The long-term safety of many antiobesity regimens has not been adequately evaluated. Unfortunately, weight gain after discontinuation of antiobesity agents is common. In addition, the effect of weight loss obtained through the use of pharmacotherapeutic agents on overall morbidity and mortality has not been established.

Like hypertension, hyperlipidemia, and diabetes, obesity should be considered a chronic medical problem that requires long-term, continuous management. As such, the treatment of obesity requires lifestyle modification. Unlike the other chronic conditions noted, a medication with proven long-term effectiveness and safety that promotes weight loss has not been developed. Antiobesity agents may be more effective in improving metabolic parameters associated with obesity rather than in achieving the desirable, ideal body weight.

REFERENCES

1. Ogden CL, Carroll MD, Curtin LR, et al. Prevalence of overweight and obesity in the United States, 1999–2004. JAMA 2006;295:1549–55.
2. Flegal KM, Graubard BI, Williamson DF, et al. Cause-specific excess deaths associated with underweight, overweight, and obesity. JAMA 2007;298:2028–37.
3. Yanovski SZ, Yanovski JA. Obesity. N Engl J Med 2002;346(8):591–602.
4. Bray GA, Greenway FL. Current and potential drugs for treatment of obesity. Endocr Rev 1999;20:805–75.
5. Cerulli J, Lomaestro BM, Malone M. Update on the pharmacotherapy of obesity. Ann Pharmacother 1998;32:88–102.
6. Carek PJ, Dickerson LM. Current concepts in the pharmacological treatment of obesity. Drugs 1999;57:883–904.
7. Dickerson LM, Carek PJ. Pharmacological treatment for obesity. Am Fam Physician 2000;61(7):2131–4.
8. Eckel RH. Nonsurgical management of obesity in adults. N Engl J Med 2008; 358(18):1941–50.

9. Anon. Diet, drugs and surgery for weight loss. Treat Guidel Med Lett 2008;6(68): 23–8.
10. Rucker D, Padwal R, Li SK, et al. Long-term pharmacotherapy for obesity and overweight: Updated meta-analysis. BMJ 2007;335:1194–9.
11. The practical guide: identification, evaluation, and treatment of overweight and obesity in adults. Bethesda (MD): National Heart, Lung, and Blood Institute/North American Association for the Study of Obesity; 2000. Available at: www.nhlbi.nih.gov/guidelines/obesity/practgde.htm. Accessed October 27, 2008.
12. Malone M. Medications associated with weight gain. Ann Pharmacother 2005;39: 2046–55.
13. Wu R-R, Zhao J-P, Jin H, et al. Lifestyle intervention and metformin for treatment of antipsychotic-induced weight gain: a randomized controlled trial. JAMA 2008; 299:185–93.
14. Bray GA. Use and abuse of appetite-suppressant drugs in the treatment of obesity. Ann Intern Med 1993;119:707–13.
15. Jung RT, Chong P. The management of obesity. Clin Endocrinol 1991;35:11–20.
16. Arner P. The β_3-adrenergic receptor - a cause and cure for obesity. N Engl J Med 1995;333:382–3.
17. Kernan WN, Viscoli CM, Brass LM, et al. Phenylpropanolamine and the risk of hemorrhagic stroke. N Engl J Med 2000;343:1826–32.
18. Bray GA. Evaluation of drugs for treating obesity. Obes Res 1995;3(Suppl 4): 425s–34s.
19. Haddock CK, Poston WS, Dill PL, et al. Pharmacotherapy for obesity: a quantitative analysis of four decades of published randomized clinical trials. Int J Obes Relat Metab Disord 2002;26:262–73.
20. Li Z, Maglione M, Wenli T, et al. Meta-analysis: pharmacological treatment of obesity. Ann Intern Med 2005;142:532–46.
21. Goldstein DJ, Potvin JH. Long-term weight loss: The effect of pharmacologic agents. Am J Clin Nutr 1994;60:647–57.
22. Weintraub M, Hasday JD, Mushlin AI, et al. A double-blind clinical trial in weight control: Use of fenfluramine and phentermine alone and in combination. Arch Intern Med 1984;144:1143–8.
23. Facts and Comparisons. Wolters Kluwer Health. Available at: www.drugfacts.com. Accessed October 28, 2008.
24. Scalfi L, D'Arrigo E, Carredente V, et al. The acute effect of dexfluramine on resting metabolic rate and post prandial thermogenesis in obese subjects: a double blind placebo controlled study. Int J Obes Relat Metab Disord 1993; 17:91–6.
25. Jick H. Heart valve disorders and appetite-suppressant drugs. JAMA 2000;283: 1738–40.
26. National Task Force on the Prevention and Treatment of Obesity. Long-term pharmacotherapy in the management of obesity. JAMA 1996;276: 1907–15.
27. Weiser M, Frishman WH, Michaelson D, et al. The pharmacologic approach to the treatment of obesity. J Clin Pharmacol 1997;37:453–73.
28. Kelly F, Jones SP, Lee IK. Sibutramine: weight loss in depressed patients. Int J Obes 1995;19(Suppl 2):145.
29. James WPT, Astrup A, Finer N, et al. Effect of sibutramine on weight maintenance after weight loss: a randomised trial. Lancet 2000;356:2119–25.
30. Bach DS, Rissanen AM, Mendel CM, et al. Absence of cardiac valve dysfunction in obese patients treated with sibutramine. Obes Res 1999;7:363–9.

31. Zannad F, Gille B, Grentzinger A, et al. Effects of sibutramine on ventricular dimensions and heart valves in obese patients during weight reduction. Am Heart J 2002;144:508–15.
32. Aronne LJ. Obesity. Med Clin North Am 1998;82(1):161–81.
33. Drent ML, van der Veen EA. Lipase inhibition: a novel concept in the treatment of obesity. Int J Obes 1993;17:241–4.
34. Drent ML, Larsson I, William-Olsson T, et al. Orlistat (Ro 18-0647), a lipase inhibitor, in the treatment of human obesity: multiple dose study. Int J Obes Relat Metab Disord 1995;19(4):221–6.
35. James WPT, Avenell A, Broom J, et al. A one-year trial to assess the value of orlistat in the management of obesity. Int J Obes 1997;21(Suppl 3):S24–30.
36. Ioannides-Demos LL, Proietto J, McNeil JJ. Pharmacotherapy for obesity. Drugs 2005;65(10):1391–418.
37. Anderson JW, Greenway FL, Fujioke K, et al. Buproprion SR enhances weight loss: a 48-week double-blind, placebo-controlled trial. Obes Res 2002;10: 633–41.
38. Chadwick DW, Marson AG. Zonisamide add-on for drug-resistant partial epilepsy. Cochrane Database Syst Rev 2003;(1):CD001416.
39. Rosenstock J, Hollander P, Gadde KM, et al. A randomized, double-blind, placebo-controlled, multicenter study to assess the efficacy and safety of topiramate controlled release in the treatment of obese type 2 diabetic patients. Diabetes Care 2007;30:1480–6.
40. Christensen R, Pernelle KK, Bartels E, et al. Efficacy and safety of the weight-loss drug rimonabant: a meta-analysis of randomized trials. Lancet 2007;370: 1706–13.

Surgical Treatment of Obesity

Megan K. Baker, MD*, T. Karl Byrne, MD, Mark E. Feldmann, MD

KEYWORDS

• Obesity • Gastric bypass • Bariatric surgery • Laparoscopy
• Nutrition

Obesity continues to be a persistently vexing problem in the United States. Obesity is defined as body mass index (BMI) greater than 30 kg/m^2, whereas morbid obesity is a BMI greater than 40 kg/m^2 or BMI greater than 35 kg/m^2 when associated with a weight-related comorbidity.[1] Patients are considered super-obese when their BMI exceeds 50 kg/m^2. Obesity-related comorbidities affect nearly every body system and include, but are not limited to, diabetes mellitus, polycystic ovarian syndrome, hypertension, hypercholesterolemia, obstructive sleep apnea, gastroesophageal reflux disease, osteoarthritis, stress urinary incontinence, depression, pseudotumor cerebri, venous stasis ulcers, and cancer. Nearly one tenth of medical expenditure in the United States can be attributed to obesity.[2]

Many treatment modalities have been developed to combat this epidemic, including surgical management. This article discusses indications for surgery, types, expectations of the surgeries, and complications a health care provider may encounter. Some of the procedures are not performed regularly anymore, but a patient may have had it previously, and primary care providers should be aware of the procedure, expectations, and long-term complications.

INDICATIONS FOR SURGERY

Treatment plans must be customized for each individual patient and should begin with the primary care provider. To be considered for surgical management, the patient must fail attempts to lose weight, such as diet, exercise, and possibly pharmacologic treatment and even complementary and alternative treatments. The patient must be psychologically stable, so a psychiatric evaluation may be necessary before referral to surgery in some situations. Any patient who has unsuccessfully attempted weight loss with a BMI greater than or equal to 40 kg/m^2 or a BMI greater than or equal to 35 kg/m^2 with a weight-related comorbidity meets criteria for referral (**Box 1**). Patients

Department of Surgery, Medical University of South Carolina, 96 Jonathan Lucas Street, Suite 420, Charleston, SC 29425, USA
* Corresponding author.
E-mail address: bakermk@musc.edu (M.K. Baker).

Prim Care Clin Office Pract 36 (2009) 417–427
doi:10.1016/j.pop.2009.01.001 **primarycare.theclinics.com**

Box 1
National Institutes of Health Consensus Panel: indications for weight loss surgery

- BMI of 40 kg/m^2 or higher
- BMI of 35 kg/m^2 or higher with a serious weight-related comorbidity
- Previous failed weight loss attempts involving an integrated nonsurgical weight loss program including dietary, behavioral, and exercise changes
- Possession of appropriate motivation and psychological stability to consent to the risk and benefits of surgery and its postoperative effects

are evaluated by the bariatric surgery team dietician and psychologist, so these referrals are not necessary before meeting with the bariatric surgery team. Any documentation of previous weight loss attempts, particularly those monitored by the primary care provider or any other practitioner, is often informative for the surgical team.

Weight loss surgery has been well documented since the mid twentieth century, and multiple procedures have been developed with varying degrees of success and risk. In 1991 the National Institutes of Health (NIH) Consensus Development Conference Panel convened and concluded that surgery was not only a viable option for weight loss in patients with a BMI of 40 kg/m^2 but in fact the most durable option. During the next 2 decades following the NIH consensus statement, the use of bariatric procedures has increased tremendously and additional procedures have been introduced. Despite these recommendations and technical improvements, less than 1% of all patients who meet criteria for weight loss surgery undergo a procedure.

BARIATRIC SURGICAL PROCEDURES

Weight loss surgery procedures typically achieve weight loss via restrictive means, malabsorptive effects, or a combination of both. Each strategy has its advantages and inherent disadvantages. Many variations of these operations exist, and some are only of historical significance now. The most commonly performed or encountered procedures are presented.

Restrictive Procedures

Gastroplasty

1. Vertical banded gastroplasty (VBG)—The VBG involves the creation of a small stomach pouch with a gastric outlet along the lesser curvature of the stomach. This outlet is buttressed by a band, restricting the gastric outlet (**Fig. 1**A).[3]
2. Adjustable gastric band (AGB)—The AGB, first developed by Kuzmak in the mid 1980s, was refined using the laparoscopic approach to the procedure now known as the laparoscopic AGB procedure (LAGB).[4] This technique achieves restriction by means of a saline-filled band, which encircles the upper portion of the stomach near the gastroesophageal junction. As more saline is injected into a subcutaneous port, more restriction to the outflow of gastric contents is achieved. LAGB has the benefit of being a low-risk, reversible, minimally invasive technique while allowing the opportunity to adjust the level of restriction with time, thereby theoretically improving long-term results (see **Fig. 1**B).
3. Sleeve gastrectomy (SG)—The laparoscopic SG, first described in 1999 as part of the biliopancreatic diversion-duodenal switch (BPD-DS) procedure, became the first of a 2-staged approach to the treatment of obesity in the super, super-obese

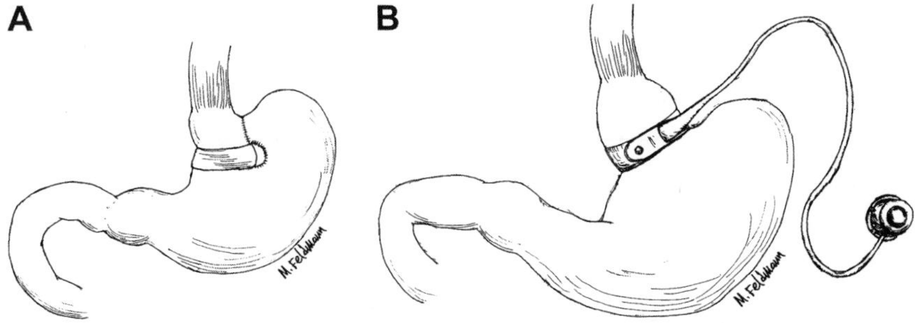

Fig. 1. (*A*) Vertical banded gastroplasty. (*B*) Laparoscopic adjustable gastric band.

category (BMI >60 kg/m^2).[5] From these procedures, significant, perhaps definitive, weight loss was noticed following the SG alone, and its use as a stand-alone procedure was proposed.[6] The technique includes resection of the majority of the antrum, body, and fundus of the stomach, leaving a lesser curve "sleeve" calibrated with a bougie or a standard endoscope.[7]

Weight loss expectations

With the technical ease and more durable success of the LAGB, the VBG has largely disappeared. Long-term data demonstrate that VBG alters postoperative eating behavior toward soft, high-calorie foods, compromising the overall weight loss achieved.[8] Conversely, the long-term Australian results for the LAGB are promising. Although LAGB patients achieve weight loss results initially less than that of the VBG, the LAGB is more durable. LAGB patients can be expected to lose 40% to 50% total excess body weight and maintain this for at least 4 years postoperatively.[9]

Results for SG are immature thus far, with only 1- to 3-year follow-up reported. Notably, though, up to 66% excess body weight loss has been reported. This is achieved via the restrictive nature of the sleeve procedure in addition to emerging hormonal mechanisms (decreased ghrelin) and increased gastric emptying.[10]

Comorbidity improvement

With resultant weight loss, weight-related comorbidities improve following LAGB. Recent data describe resolution of diabetes mellitus in 47.9%, hypertension in 43.2%, hyperlipidemia in 58.9%, and obstructive sleep apnea in 95% of patients undergoing LAGB.[11] Further, this success appears to be durable up to 6 years postoperative as demonstrated in European studies.[12] No long-term data are currently available on comorbidity resolution with SG.

Malabsorptive Procedures

Malabsorptive procedures were mainly used in the mid twentieth century. Initially, the jejunoileal bypass was most commonly performed, but due to its severe associated malabsorption with protein-calorie and vitamin deficiencies, the procedure fell into disfavor. These procedures were further refined in the 1970s to the biliopancreatic diversion (BPD) and subsequently complemented with the BPD-DS (**Fig. 2**A, B). The BPD achieves its weight loss via acceleration in both gastric emptying (via gastrectomy) and intestinal transit time (via enteroileostomy). Many variations of this procedure have been used, all of which vary in the extent of the gastrectomy performed and the length of the common enteric channel developed by the enteroileostomy.[13]

Table 1
Long-term follow-up after bariatric surgery

	Evaluation Visits (with Surgeon)	Laboratory Evaluation	Weight Loss Expected
Restrictive procedures	6–12 visits per year for 2–3 y, then annually, or as indicated by loss of dietary restriction or weight regain	As directed by comorbidities	LAGB 40%–50% excess SG up to 66% of excess VBG 50% of excess (not enduring)
Malabsorptive procedures	1, 3, 6, 12, and 18 mo postoperatively, then annually for life	CBC, BMP, prealbumin, albumin, total protein, folate, iron, thiamin, vitamin B12, calcium, 25-hydroxy vitamin D; a as directed by comorbidities	BPD±DS more than 70% of excess
Combination	1, 3, 6, 12, and 18 mo postoperatively, then annually for life	CBC, BMP, prealbumin, albumin, total protein, folate, Iron, thiamin, vitamin B12, calcium, 25-hydroxy vitamin D; a as directed by comorbidities	57%–68% of excess

Abbreviations: BMP, basic metabolic panel; CBC, complete blood count.

The most widely used variation though is the addition of a DS procedure. In the BPD-DS, an SG is performed, and the duodenum is divided just distal to the pylorus. This affords the patient the sensation of early satiety and reduces the parietal cell mass, rendering improved weight loss and fewer problems with marginal ulceration, respectively.[14]

Weight loss expectation

BPD ± DS achieves excellent sustainable weight loss. In a series of more than 400 patients, Hess and Hess noted more than 70% excess body weight loss with 8 years of follow-up (**Table 1**).[14] Importantly, when compared with the Roux-en-Y gastric bypass (RYGB) (both a restrictive and malabsorptive operation), the BPD has been found to achieve significantly greater weight loss in the super-obese population.[15] Although quite effective at achieving significant weight loss, the perioperative complication rate renders this less desirable in patients with BMIs below 60 kg/m^2.

Comorbidity improvement

Like overall weight loss rates, patients' comorbidities dramatically improve following BPD-DS. In a recent meta-analysis, 98.8% of diabetic patients had complete remission of their diabetes, whereas 83% of BPD-DS patients with hypertension experienced resolution of their high blood pressure. Improvements also included resolution of hyperlipidemia (99.9%), hypertriglyceridemia (100%), and sleep apnea (71.2%).[11]

Combination Malabsorptive and Restrictive Procedures

The gastric bypass procedure, first described by Mason and Ito[16] in the mid 1960s, consists of a small restrictive gastric pouch, which is anastamosed to a loop of jejunum. The modernized version involves the creation of a 20 to 30 cc pouch, complete division of the pouch from the excluded stomach, which remains in vivo,

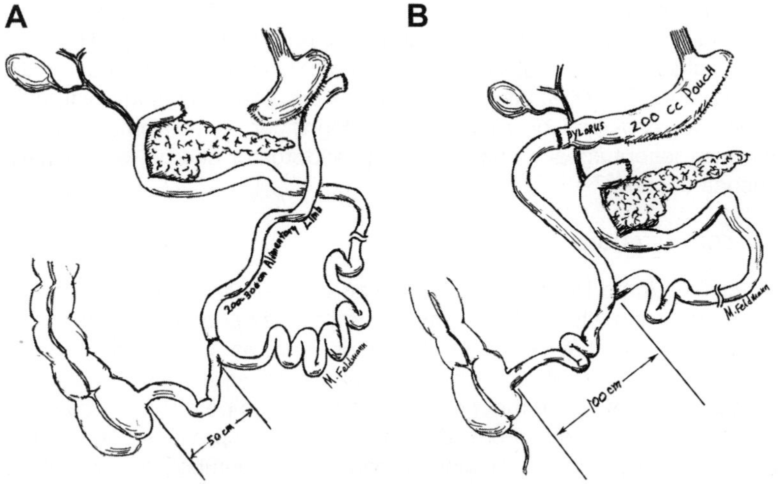

Fig. 2. (*A*) biliopancreatic diversion. (*B*) Biliopancreatic diversion with duodenal switch.

and anastomosis of the pouch to the jejunum using an RYGB formation (**Fig. 3**). The length of the Roux-en-Y limb varies depending on the patient's BMI. Like BPD-DS, this technique has been entirely adapted and further refined using a laparoscopic approach.[17]

Weight loss expectation

Either approach to RYGB achieves significant weight loss, ranging from 57% to 68% excess body weight at 1 year (see **Table 1**).[18]

Comorbidity improvement

Most patients diagnosed preoperatively with metabolic syndrome (combination of hypertension, dyslipidemia, glucose intolerance, and obesity) experience reversal of their condition within the first postoperative year following RYGB.[19,20] Buchwald's

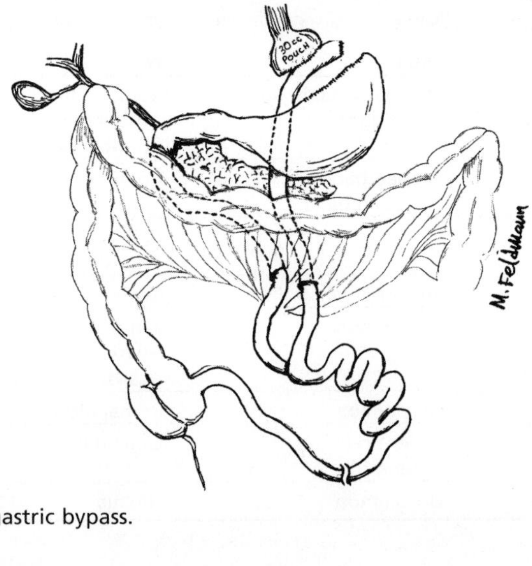

Fig. 3. Roux-en-Y gastric bypass.

meta-analysis of more than 136 studies including 22,000 patients summarizes the improvement in comorbidities after RYGB as follows: improvement in Hgb A1C levels and fasting glucose levels (83%), complete resolution of hypertension (67.5%) and improvement in up to 87%, improved hyperlipidemia (96.9%), and obstructive sleep apnea (94.8% resolution or improvement). Significant improvement in conditions such as gastroesophageal reflux disease, pseudotumor cerebri, and urinary stress incontinence occurs.[11]

SURGICAL COMPLICATIONS

Complications related to bariatric surgery can occur at any time, but they fall into 2 categories, early and late. Patients may present to their primary care doctor or emergency department before seeing their surgeon, and, as such, a familiarity with the signs and symptoms seen with common complications is helpful. Descriptions of complications related to the most common procedures performed today have been provided and are summarized based on symptoms and presentation in **Table 2**. To minimize 1 postsurgical complication, venous thromboembolism prophylaxis using low-molecular weight heparin is indicated in most patients.[21]

Restrictive Procedures

Both VBG and LAGB are associated with postoperative complications. The VBG has greater acute morbidity than that of the LAGB, whereas the latter suffers from a higher reoperation rate. Complications of the VBG include stomal stenosis, which may be intractable, reflux esophagitis, pouch and esophageal dilation, and ultimately weight regain, especially in sweets eaters. Unlike the VBG, the LAGB is better tolerated early on, but as seen in a large European trial, more than 20% of LAGB patients require reoperation for complications, such as band slippage, band erosion, port and port-tubing fractures or flips, pouch dilation, and port-site infection with time.[22,23] Refinements in the technique to place the band have been made to diminish the incidence of band slippage. Both the VBG and LAGB are associated with very low mortality, 0.5% and 0.05%, respectively.[9]

Table 2
Signs and symptoms of complications after common bariatric procedures

	LAGB	RYGB
Nausea/vomiting	Slipped band, band too tight	Stomal stenosis, internal hernia (patient may have benign abdominal examination)
Abdominal pain	Slipped band, eroded band	Stomal ulcer, internal hernia
Fever, tachycardia	Port-site infection	Early postoperative period → anastomotic leak
Shortness of breath	Pulmonary embolism	Pulmonary embolism
Diarrhea	Uncommon	Dumping syndrome (noncompliance with diet, ingestion of simple carbohydrates)
Melena	Uncommon	Stomal ulcer
Weight regain	Patient requires band fill	Noncompliance with diet
Fatigue	Uncommon	Anemia

Mortality associated with SG is 0.6%. Complications are also low and include risk of leak(0.9%), pulmonary embolus (0.3%), reoperation (4.5%), and wound infection (0.1%).[7]

Malabsorptive Procedures

Malabsorptive procedures were historically plagued by their associated nutritional deficiencies. Specifically, as detailed in Scopinaro's 20-year experience with BPD, calcium deficiency, anemia, protein malnutrition, and thiamine deficiencies are common.[24] However, most of these abnormalities can be prevented via postoperative lifelong supplementation of calcium, iron, folate, thiamine, vitamin B12, and fat-soluble vitamins. Protein malabsorption can be positively affected by the length of the common channel created at the time of the initial operation so as to increase nutrient absorption. BPD-associated mortality rates have been low, ranging from 0% to 1.9%. The most common surgical complications include incisional hernia (18%) and anastomotic ulcer (6.3%–10%).[14,25] Additionally, patients who undergo a BPD-DS using a laparoscopic technique experience fewer wound-related complications.[25] Commonly, the BPD may be passed over in lieu of other combination procedures to the degree of protein malabsorption described.

Combination Procedure

Complications related to both open and laparoscopic RYGB have historically remained low but differ slightly depending on the technique used. Both the open and laparoscopic approach are associated with a risk of pulmonary embolus (0.78%) and anastomotic leak (1.68%).[26] The risk of anastomotic leak in the laparoscopic setting does appear to be related to the surgeon's learning curve, decreasing with growing surgeon experience.[27,28] When compared with the open approach, the laparoscopic RYGB does afford a significant reduction in the risk of incisional hernia (24% vs 11%) but a slight increase in the risk of marginal ulceration, stomal stenosis, and internal hernia.[29,30]

RYGB is often associated with dumping syndrome (85% of patients). BPD can also result in dumping by virtue of the anatomic alterations, but it is not as commonly seen as that in RYGB. The symptoms range from mild to severe and are usually related to poor food choices. The condition is related to the ingestion of refined sugars or high-glycemic carbohydrates. When this occurs, symptoms can present in their early form (30–60 minutes after eating: sweating, flushing, tachycardia, palpitations, diarrhea, cramping) or later (1–3 hours after eating: sweating, shakiness, fainting, loss of concentration). Early symptoms result from the rapid emptying of sugars from the gastric pouch, which results in a release of gut hormones, whereas late symptoms result from hypoglycemia. Either of these can be prevented by simply avoiding these foods.[31] No workup is necessary if patients present with these classic symptoms, which resolve when they comply with proper dietary recommendations.

The issue of internal hernia following RYGB warrants special attention. Patients who have undergone this procedure are at lifelong risk for internal herniation of their intestinal contents. Although this is uncommon, if an internal hernia is not corrected, an abdominal catastrophe can ensue.[32] This diagnosis is very difficult to make and may require operative exploration to do so. If an RYGB patient presents with abdominal pain with or without nausea and vomiting, the diagnosis must be entertained. Patients will often have a benign abdominal examination and may have only subtle findings, if any, on computed tomographic scan. Plain abdominal radiographs are not particularly helpful. If pain persists and the remainder of the workup has proven negative, then operative exploration is warranted.[32]

LONG-TERM FOLLOW-UP AFTER BARIATRIC SURGERY

Follow-Up and Nutrition

Success following any type of bariatric surgery depends largely on long-term follow-up. Several issues must be surveyed for and addressed during the postoperative period, which include the following: weight loss, weight-related comorbidities, nutrition, and potential surgical complications. This approach helps to ensure maximal weight loss, prevention of weight regain, avoidance of nutritional deficiencies, and prompt recognition of any surgery-related complications.

The frequency of follow-up will be directly related to the type of surgical procedure that patients undergo. For example, patients who undergo an LAGB are evaluated by their surgical team monthly for the first 2 years, as adjustments are needed for their band. Patients who undergo malabsorptive procedures are followed both clinically and with nutritional assessment quarterly for the first year, semiannually for the second postoperative year, and annually thereafter by their surgeon.

The nutritional evaluation will differ depending on the nature of the procedure. For patients undergoing purely restrictive procedures, laboratory monitoring is indicated as related to the patients' comorbidities. In contrast, patients who undergo malabsorptive procedures will require laboratory evaluation surveying for vitamin deficiency (vitamin B12, folate, thiamin, vitamin D), mineral deficiency (calcium), protein malnutrition (prealbumin, albumin, total protein), anemia (complete blood count [CBC], iron), and dehydration/electrolyte abnormality (basic metabolic panel [BMP]) (see **Table 2**). Patients who have an RYGB will require supplementation in excess of a traditional multivitamin. Given the malabsorptive nature of the procedure, fat-soluble vitamins and calcium are at particular risk of becoming deficient. Notably, calcium citrate is much better absorbed and recommended over calcium gluconate in this population.[33,34] The recommended supplementation is listed in **Box 2**. Ideally, patients should be followed by their bariatric surgical team; but for those patients who are not able or willing to, referral to a dietician familiar with weight loss surgery is required only if derangements in their laboratory evaluation exist.

SUMMARY

Morbid obesity is a disease that is effectively treated with surgery. The ideal treatment for the disease would be prevention; however, given the epidemic of obesity in the United States, we will likely be required to continue a multidisciplinary approach to the treatment of morbid obesity. Treatment plans must be customized for each individual patient and should involve evaluation by the primary care provider, a dietician,

Box 2
Recommended daily nutritional supplementation following Roux-en-Y gastric bypass[36]

- Multivitamin—(200% of daily value, at least 18 mg iron, 400 μg folic acid, selenium, and zinc)
- Vitamin B12—350–500 μg/d orally
- Calcium citrate with Vitamin D3—1500–2000 mg/d
- Elemental iron—18–27 mg/d
- B complex—1/d

Data from Aills L, Blankenship J, Buffington C, et al. ASMBS Allied Health nutritional guidelines for the surgical weight loss patient. Surg Obes Relat Dis 2008;4(Suppl 5):S73–108.

Table 3
Key practice recommendations

Clinical Recommendation	Evidence Rating	Reference
Bariatric surgery leads to sustainable long-term weight loss	A	11
Bariatric surgery leads to significant reduction or resolution of weight-related diabetes mellitus, hypertension, and dyslipidemia	A	11
Venous thromboembolism prophylaxis using low-molecular weight heparin is indicated in most patients	A	21
Patients should be evaluated in a multidisciplinary manner to include medical, psychological, nutritional, and surgical evaluation	C	35

psychologist, and surgeon. Then, depending on the patient's individual needs, comorbidities, and candidacy, a surgical plan is determined.

Short-term weight loss is greatest with the BPD-DS approach, but it is also associated with higher complications. This may be justified in patients who are super-morbidly obese. Both the LAGB and the RYGB have long-term data establishing their efficacy in all patient groups and should be considered early in a patient's course before the development of significant sequelae from comorbidities (**Table 3**). With any procedure, lifelong follow-up is mandatory, as these patients will require monitoring for nutritional assessment, weight maintenance, and surveillance for complications.

REFERENCES

1. Panel NIoHCDC. Gastrointestinal surgery for severe obesity. Ann Intern Med 1991;115:956–91.
2. Finkelstein E, Fiebelkorn IC, Wang G. National medical spending attributable to overweight and obesity: how much, and who's paying? Health Aff 2003;12(1):18–24.
3. Buchwald HB, Buchwald JN. Evolution of operative procedures for the management of morbid obesity 1950–2000. Obes Surg 2002;12:705–17.
4. LK. Silicone gastric banding: a simple and effective operation for morbid obesity. Contemp Surg 1986;28:13–8.
5. Gumbs AA, Gagner M, Dakin G, et al. Sleeve gastrectomy for morbid obesity. Obes Surg 1999;17:962–9.
6. Deitel M, Crosby RD, Gagner M. The first international consensus summit for sleeve gastrectomy (SG), New York City, October 25–27, 2007. Obes Surg 2008;18:487–96.
7. Akkary E, Duffy A, Bell R. Deciphering the sleeve: technique, indications, efficacy and safety of sleeve gastrectomy. Obes Surg 2008;18(10):1329–39.
8. Brolin RL, Robertson LB, Kenler HA, et al. Weight loss and dietary intake after vertical banded gastroplasty and Roux-en-Y gastric bypass. Ann Surg 1994;220(6):782–90.
9. Chapman AE, Kiroff G, Game P, et al. Laparoscopic adjustable gastric banding in the treatment of obesity: a systematic literature review. Surgery 2004;135(3):326–51.

10. Himpens J, Dapri G, Cadiere GB. A prospective randomized study between laparoscopic gastric banding and laparoscopic isolated sleeve gastrectomy: results after 1 and 3 years. Obes Surg 2006;16:1450–6.
11. Buchwald H, Avidor Y, Braunwald E, et al. Bariatric surgery: a systematic review and metaanalysis. JAMA 2004;292(14):1724–37.
12. Mittermair RP, Aigner F, Nehoda H, et al. Laparoscopic Swedish adjustable gastric banding: 6-year follow-up and comparison to other laparoscopic bariatric procedures. Obes Surg 2003;13:412–7.
13. Van Hee H. Biliopancreatic diversion in the surgical treatment of morbid obesity. World J Surg 2004;28:435–44.
14. Hess DS, Hess DW. Biliopancreatic diversion with duodenal switch. Obes Surg 1998;8:267–82.
15. Brolin RE, Kenler HA, Gorman JH, et al. Long-limb gastric bypass in the superobese. A prospective randomized study. Ann Surg 1992;215(4):387–95.
16. Mason EE, Ito C. Gastric bypass in obesity, 1967. Obes Res 1996;4(3):316–9.
17. Whitgrove AC, clark GW. Laparoscopic gastric bypass. Roux en-Y 500 patients: technique and results, with 3–60 month follow-up. Obes Surg 2000;10:233–9.
18. Perugini RA, Mason R, Czerniach DR, et al. Predictors of complication and suboptimal weight loss after laparoscopic roux-en-Y gastric bypass: a series of 188 patients. Arch Surg 2003;138:541–6.
19. Sugerman HJ, Wolfe LG, Sica DA, et al. Diabetes and hypertension in severe obesity and effects of gastric bypass induced weight loss. Ann Surg 2003; 237(6):751–8.
20. Lee WJ, Huang MT, Wang W, et al. Effects of obesity surgery on the metabolic syndrome. Arch Surg 2004;139:1088–92.
21. Geerts WH, Pineo GF, Heit JA, et al. Prevention of venous thromboembolism: the Seventh ACCP Conference on antithrombotic and thrombolytic therapy. Chest 2004;126(Suppl 3):S338–400.
22. Belachew M, Belva PH, Desaive C. Long-term results of laparoscopic adjustable gastric banding for the treatment of morbid obesity. Obes Surg 2002;12(4): 564–8.
23. Martikainen T, Pirinen E, Alhava E, et al. Long-term results, late complications and quality of life in a series of adjustable gastric banding. Obes Surg 2004;14:648–54.
24. Scopinaro N, Adami GF, Marinari GM, et al. Biliopancreatic diversion. World J Surg 1998;22:936–46.
25. Kim WW, Gagner M, Kini S, et al. Laparoscopic vs. open biliopancreatic diversion with duodenal switch: a case series of 40 consecutive patients. J Gastrointest Surg 2003;7(4):552–7.
26. Podnos YD, jimenez JC, Wilson SE, et al. Complications after laparoscopic gastric bypass: a review of 3464 cases. Arch Surg 2003;138:957–61.
27. Schauer P, Ikramuddin S, Gourash W, et al. Outcomes after laparoscopic roux-en-y gastric bypass in 100 cases. Ann Surg 2000;232(4):515–29.
28. Schauer P, Idramuddin S, Hamad G, et al. The learning curve for laparoscopic Roux-en-Y gastric bypass in 100 cases. Surg Endosc 2003;17:212–5.
29. Fernandez AZ, DeMaria EJ, Tichansky DS, et al. Experience with over 3,000 open and laparoscopic bariatric procedures: multivariate analysis of factors related to leak and resultant mortality. Surg Endosc 2004;18:193–7.
30. Nguyen NT, Goldman C, Rosenquist CJ, et al. Laparoscopic versus open gastric bypass: a randomized study of outcomes, quality of life, and costs. Ann Surg 2001;234(2):279–89 [discussion: 289–91].

31. American Society for Metabolic and Bariatric Surgery (ASBS) Public/Professional Education Committee. Bariatric surgery: postoperative concerns. Revised February 7, 2008. Available at: http://www.asbs.org/html/pdf/asbs_bspc.pdf. Accessed April 15, 2009.
32. Pitt T, Brethauer S, Sherman V, et al. Diagnostic laparoscopy for chronic abdominal pain after gastric bypass. Surg Obes Relat Dis 2008;3:394–8 [discussion: 398].
33. Gasteyger C, Suter M, Gaillard RC, et al. Nutritional deficiencies after Roux-en-Y gastric bypass for morbid obesity often cannot be prevented by standard multivitamin supplementation. Am J Clin Nutr 2008;87(5):1128–33.
34. Coupaye M, Puchaux K, Bogard C, et al. Nutritional consequences of adjustable gastric banding and gastric bypass: a 1-year prospective study. Obes Res 2009; 19(1):56–65.
35. Buchwald H. Consensus Conference Statement: bariatric surgery for morbid obesity. Health implications for patients, health professionals and third-party payers. Surg Obes Relat Dis 2005;1:371–81.
36. Aills L, Blankenship J, Buffinington C, et al. ASMBS Allied Health nutritional guidelines for the surgical weight loss patient. Surg Obes Relat Dis 2008;4(suppl 5): s73–108.

Index

Note: Page numbers of article titles are in **boldface** type.

Prim Care Clin Office Pract 36 (2009) 429–438
doi:10.1016/S0095-4543(09)00046-3 **primarycare.theclinics.com**

D

E

M

N

Q

R

S